Pain Psychology for Clinicians

Pain Psychology for Clinicians

A Practical Guide for the Non-Psychologist Managing Patients with Chronic Pain

Leanne R. Cianfrini, PhD

Registered Psychologist
Pain and Medication Management Program
CBI Health Group
Abbotsford, BC, Canada

Elizabeth J. Richardson, PhD, MSPH

Assistant Professor
Behavioral and Social Sciences
University of Montevallo
Montevallo, AL, USA

Daniel M. Doleys, PhD

Director
Doleys Clinic/Pain and Rehabilitation Institute
Birmingham, AL, USA

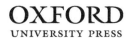

OXFORD
UNIVERSITY PRESS

OXFORD
UNIVERSITY PRESS

Oxford University Press is a department of the University of Oxford. It furthers
the University's objective of excellence in research, scholarship, and education
by publishing worldwide. Oxford is a registered trade mark of Oxford University
Press in the UK and certain other countries.

Published in the United States of America by Oxford University Press
198 Madison Avenue, New York, NY 10016, United States of America.

Library of Congress Cataloging-in-Publication Data
Names: Cianfrini, Leanne R., author. | Richardson, Elizabeth J. author. |
Doleys, Daniel M., author.
Title: Pain psychology for clinicians : a practical guide for the
non-psychologist managing patients with chronic pain /
Leanne R. Cianfrini, Elizabeth J. Richardson, Daniel M. Doleys.
Description: New York, NY : Oxford University Press, [2021] |
Includes bibliographical references and index.
Identifiers: LCCN 2020039400 (print) | LCCN 2020039401 (ebook) |
ISBN 9780197504727 (paperback) | ISBN 9780197504741 (epub) |
ISBN 9780197504758
Subjects: MESH: Pain Management—methods | Chronic Pain—psychology |
Primary Health Care | Physician-Patient Relations
Classification: LCC RB127 (print) | LCC RB127 (ebook) | NLM WL 704.6 |
DDC 616/.0472—dc23
LC record available at https://lccn.loc.gov/2020039400
LC ebook record available at https://lccn.loc.gov/2020039401

DOI: 10.1093/med/9780197504727.001.0001

1 3 5 7 9 8 6 4 2

Printed by Marquis, Canada

Contents

Preface

Estimates suggest that 50 to 100 million persons in the United States suffer from some kind of chronic pain condition. There is no indication that the prevalence or incidence is decreasing with time. Indeed, the number of hospital admissions for children complaining of pain is increasing. Chronic pain has finally come to be recognized as a disease process, not unlike diabetes and hypertension. In many instances, this persistent pain will require life-long management. The situation is further complicated when one recognizes that chronic pain can be a component of other diseases. The availability of trained pain management specialists prepared to work collaboratively with patients over the long haul is sadly wanting, with the majority of pain clinics offering unidimensional short-term interventions rather than interdisciplinary care models that promote lasting self-management tools.

Many patients with chronic pain present to primary care settings. Their situations can be very complex, shrouded in a number of physical and psychosocial factors. The time and resources needed to effectively manage this group of patients are rarely available. Already overburdened clinicians can only do the best they can. Often, this means taking an almost palliative approach, with an emphasis on maintenance of the best quality of life possible with little expectation of significant improvement. Working in this arena can be frustrating and emotionally taxing on the patients, clinicians, and staff.

This book is designed to provide some meaningful communication approaches to the management of the patient with chronic pain, whether it is the primary complaint or secondary to another disease process. It is no secret that the clinician–patient therapeutic relationship is the bedrock of effective management. Patients may come seeking your reassurance and understanding. Based on past medical experiences, they may feel they have something to prove or defend. They may take a passive approach to recommended treatment plans. They may be fearful of the pain and expect you to guide them. They may have concerning behaviors surrounding opioid use. They may be suffering from comorbid mood disorders that complicate the symptom presentation. They may exhibit unrealistic expectations or angry and challenging attitudes. Understanding the psychological nuances of office-based interactions can help to ease frustration and improve care.

Combined, the authors have more than 70 years of experience treating patients with chronic pain in community-based settings from a behavioral medicine perspective. At one point or another, they have encountered every clinical vignette described herein. This is not intended to be an academic or theoretical book, but rather a practical guide to communication strategies based on research evidence—a "speak like a pain psychologist" primer, if you will. No doubt some readers of this book will already possess a good deal of insight and skillful communication abilities. We hope they will find the suggestions presented here a positive reinforcement of their skills and efforts. The intent is not to provide the "nuts and bolts" specifics on how to treat chronic pain, how to use opioid therapy, or how to treat pain-related mood disorders. Those topics are covered well in other workbooks and textbooks. Rather, the information is offered as a reminder that simple communication strategies that convey both empathy and expertise can go a long way toward creating positive functional outcomes, enhancing patient satisfaction, and restoring meaning and value in a challenging clinical career.

LRC, EJR, and, DMD

About the Authors

Leanne R. Cianfrini, PhD, is a registered psychologist with the CBI Health Group Abbotsford Pain and Medication Management Program in British Columbia, Canada. She has served on various committees for the American Academy of Pain Medicine and Alabama Psychological Association. She is Past President of the Southern Pain Society. As an Adjunct Assistant Professor at UAB, she taught the core graduate-level Intervention and Behavioral Observation course for over 10 years. Her clinical orientations and interests include Cognitive Behavioral Therapy for pain and insomnia, Acceptance and Commitment Therapy, motivational interviewing for health promotion and relapse prevention, brief solutions-focused therapy, and mindfulness training.

Elizabeth J. Richardson, PhD, MSPH, is Assistant Professor of Social and Behavioral Sciences at the University of Montevallo, teaching a variety of courses including the Psychology of Pain. Dr. Richardson's specialty in clinical psychology is working with individuals who have chronic pain and has served as pain psychologist for a comprehensive pain rehabilitation program with the Department of Veteran's Affairs. Her research focuses pain perception, chronic pain, psychological treatments for pain, spinal cord injury, and the interrelationships among health, biology, the brain, and behavior.

Daniel M. Doleys, PhD, is the Director of The Doleys Clinic/Pain and Rehabilitation Institute in Birmingham, Alabama. Prior to starting in private practice, he was an Associate Professor of Psychology in the School of Medicine at the University of Alabama, Birmingham. His clinical and research interests have focused on the assessment and treatment of chronic pain. He is the recipient of the Distinguished Research Psychologist Award from the Alabama Psychological Association, as well as the Excellence in Research and Clinical Care Award, the Distinguished Service Award, and the Dr. Hubert L. and Renee S. Rosomoff Award for Excellence in Pain from the from the Southern Pain Society.

1
Why Introduce Psychological Techniques into Clinical Practice?

Daniel M. Doleys

Think back to your schedule over the past few weeks. Were there any days where you reviewed the list of upcoming appointments and muttered something to the effect of, "Do I really have to see *him* today? Nothing ever gets accomplished. He is never happy." Were there any days you felt like passing along a particular patient to a colleague as you were simply "not in the mood" to deal with her? How do you feel about the patient who verbally blocks your departure from the exam room with, "Please, I have just *one more* small thing." What about the patient who winces and moans and clutches in pain if you even get close to the table to perform an exam, or the patient who says with no remorse, "I had to take more hydrocodone because I was hurting more this month. You *need* to give me an early refill." Sometimes, Friday afternoons can't come fast enough and Monday mornings arrive way too fast. Clinical practice would be so much easier if all we had to do was follow our evidence-based medical algorithms—without dealing with the patient.

Of course, the above is somewhat tongue-in-cheek, but the emotional stress of patient care and caregiving is well documented and has long been recognized.[1,2] The effects can impact the clinician personally and professionally: personal health, family dynamics, mood, and work satisfaction are all vulnerable. O'Dowd,[3] highlighting how a certain type of patient can affect the clinician, used the adjective "heartsink" in reference to patients who "exasperate, defeat, and overwhelm their doctors by their behavior. While heartsink patients often have serious medical problems, they are a disparate group of individuals whose only common thread seems to be the distress they cause their doctor and the practice" (p. 528). The patient's problems and presentation seem impenetrable.

If you're reading this book, chances are you have also chosen, intentionally or not, to work with one of the most complicated conditions—chronic pain. Chronic pain and pain-related diagnoses, such as osteoarthritis, degenerative disc disease, or fibromyalgia, are among the top few reasons patients visit their primary care physician.[4] Chronic pain is a challenge for health care practitioners on the front lines of clinical service delivery, in part because the very definition specifies the presence and complex interplay of both somatic and emotional components.[5] Chronic pain itself is recognized as a disease process by many,[6,7] but it lacks clear objective biomarkers at this time. Although efforts aimed at elucidating functional brain imaging signatures and genetic biomarkers are under way,[8,9] current practitioners are compelled to consider and attend almost exclusively to the patient's subjective reports. As we know, diagnostic scans like x-rays and magnetic resonance imaging (MRI) may discover structural injury or pathology, but they are not accurate proxies for the patient's individual pain experience.

Laboratory studies and clinical trials necessarily separate out homogenous groups to examine individual differences in the pain experience or to determine effective treatments. However, in practice, patients present with complex and dynamic biopsychological complaints within their unique cultural perspective. Our clinic days involve a quite heterogenous and diverse group of patients with unpredictable courses, influences that extend back to childhood, and a host of contributing medical and psychological comorbidities. Scott-Warren[10] expressed this experience as

> Every patient ... almost without exception, is enshrouded in a multifarious, intricate interplay of the biological, psychological, and social ... that collectively precipitate the situations in which individuals burdened with chronic pain find themselves. As such, the comorbidities ... include diverse conditions such as depression, hypertension, catastrophizing, insomnia, and obesity to name a few." (p. 888)

Some 70% of individuals living with chronic pain also have been diagnosed with a psychiatric/psychological disorder. The incidence of comorbid depression has ranged up to 85%.[11] Furthermore, the extensive use of opioids as part of pain management has significantly changed the landscape of problematic situations faced by clinicians. One study of primary care practices uncovered an opioid use disorder in 30% of patients.[12] Thus, effective treatment of the patient with the disease of chronic pain takes on an entirely new dimension, one that necessitates the inclusion of psychological principles and techniques. Psychology plays a role in at least three broad areas:

1. Uncovering and treating psychosocial factors that contribute to the patient's individual experience of and treatment outcomes for chronic pain
2. Recognizing the clinician's predilections and biases brought to patient interactions and treatment decisions
3. Enhancing communication between the clinician and patient.

It is easy to understand how caring for the chronic pain patient can place significant demands on the clinician and require an arsenal of communication techniques and skills.

Purpose and Structure of This Book

Throughout the book, we will use the generic term *clinician*. It is intended to encompass a variety of medical personnel, including physicians, physician assistants (PAs), and certified registered nurse practitioners (CRNPs). However, the information is applicable to any professional or trainee participating in the care of the patient with chronic pain.

The purpose behind this book is to provide a variety of efficient, realistic skills and techniques to help clinicians in their routine communication with chronic pain patients. Other books have presented detailed overviews of contemporary psychological approaches to pain management (see the Further Reading section at the end of the chapter). Chapter 2 summarizes these approaches to provide background to support our patient scenario chapters. Vignettes ("Cases") for most commonly encountered challenges in clinical practice will be used to demonstrate how to effectively incorporate key concepts from well-established psychological therapies such as cognitive–behavioral therapy (CBT), acceptance and commitment therapy (ACT), and motivational interviewing (MI) into the clinical setting. We will present background research to support recommendations for brief clinical interventions ("Context") and suggest practical solutions to enhance conversations with patients ("Communication"). Although these therapies in full can be time-consuming and are designed to be used by trained psychological professionals, components can be adapted and streamlined for use by any clinician in the medical office–based practice.

Acquiring and implementing some basic, but evidence-based, techniques can save time and emotional energy as well as enhance patient outcomes. Emphasis is placed on sharing the burden of responsibility for effective treatment with patients and moving them toward self-management, including the use of interdisciplinary modalities. This is not unlike the model for treating diabetes wherein diet, nutrition, weight management, and exercise become key components of long-term management. Helping the patient understand chronic pain as a similar disease process requiring a longitudinal and team approach to its management is an important foundation. Although technical knowledge in medical practice may be our comfort zone, and the age of electronic medical records seems to reduce the patient's symptom experience to a series of click-boxes, we should not underestimate the therapeutic power of language, active listening, and empathic human interaction.

Another important aspect of this book is to help clinicians determine when the complexity of the patient is such that referral to a multidisciplinary pain clinic/psychiatrist/addiction recovery center should be considered. This book is designed to help clinicians recognize the emotions and motivations driving both their part and the patient's part of the clinical interaction, but it is not intended to replace psychotherapy or appropriate counseling referrals. Clinicians must be able to recognize the limits of their background, training, and practice.

The Role of Psychology and Pain Psychologists

Pain psychology has emerged as an area of study and practice in its own right. The notion has long been displaced that somatic pain symptoms are simply a manifestation of "psychogenic pain"; that antiquated model implicated some unidentified maladaptive psychological/psychiatric force as the causal and perpetuating factor for pain. Instead, there is a recognition that psychological variables, including mood states, expectations, inherent and taught coping skills, quality of patient–clinician interactions, and other variables, can significantly impact the experience of pain as well as treatment outcomes. In a word, pain can best be addressed within its biopsychosocial context. While pain psychologists have been instrumental in the development of theories and therapies, anyone interacting and communicating with the patient is going to engage in some level of "pain psychology," intentionally or subconsciously. Clinically, it is important to understand and make explicit the nuances of these interactions so they can be used to the best advantage of clinician and patient.

Pain psychologists are a unique group of clinicians. They generally hold a doctoral degree in psychology and are licensed by a local or regional agency to practice psychology. This requires possessing appropriate credentials and passing national and state licensing exams. Many have completed a fellowship and are usually active in regional and national pain-related organizations, most of which are interdisciplinary in nature. Pain psychologists may practice in an academic setting, a hospital, a primary care office, an outpatient pain management clinic, or an individual or group private psychotherapy practice. Although identified as clinical psychologists, many have extensive training and knowledge in areas such as anatomy, neurophysiology, pharmacology, and genetics as they relate to pain and pain processing. They are familiar with a broad range of medically based pain therapies (e.g., interventional procedures, neuromodulation, medications). More importantly, they recognize how psychological factors can influence the outcome of these therapies.

Some pain psychologists devote a large percentage of their time to research. Volumes of high-quality research involving well-controlled studies have demonstrated the contribution of psychological variables and help to drive clinical practice standards. For example, research in the field of chronic pain has demonstrated the impact of perceived consequences,[13] mood,[14] gender of the experimenter/observer,[15] presence of a reinforcing spouse,[16] and knowledge of neurophysiology[17] on pain ratings provided by subjects in experimental situations. Table 1.1 summarizes other psychological variables and their effects on pain and function that have been subjected to systematic study. Examples of treatment strategies that have been used to influence the effects of these variables are also given.

In the clinical setting, psychologists perform a variety of important functions. Almost every national or state guideline and administrative code relating to the use of chronic opioid therapy recommends a risk assessment addressing the likelihood that a patient may not be safe and compliant with prescribed controlled substances. Rather than attempting to identify the "bad

Table 1.1 Psychological variables that influence pain and function

Psychological Variable	Description	Impact on Pain and Function	Treatment Strategies
Attention and pain salience	Pain captures and diverts our attention.	• Increased vigilance and anticipation can increase pain intensity. • Distraction can decrease pain intensity.	• Distraction techniques • Interoceptive exposure • Mindfulness techniques
Cognitions/ beliefs	Thoughts and beliefs influence pain intensity and function.	• Interpretation and beliefs affect pain. • Catastrophizing and negative thoughts can increase pain and disability. • Expectations influence outcomes, pain, and function.	• Psychoeducation • Cognitive restructuring • CBT
Emotional reactivity	Negative emotions associated with pain can influence pain intensity, cognitions, attention, and functioning.	• Fear, anxiety, depression, and distress can increase pain and activity avoidance.	• CBT • ACT • Mindfulness-based stress reduction • Behavioral activation to increase exposure to positive experiences
Pain behaviors	The manner in which one copes with pain, in turn, influences pain perception.	• Escape/avoidance behaviors can increase disability and distress. • Lack of pacing (under- or over-activity) can promote pain. • Overt behaviors inadvertently communicate pain to others.	• Operant conditioning techniques (e.g., reinforcing desired behavior) • In vivo exposure therapy such as desensitization/ gradual exposure to exercises and activities • Coping skills training

Table 1.1 *Continued*

Psychological Variable	Description	Impact on Pain and Function	Treatment Strategies
Dependence/ overreliance on medical-based treatments	Defers to medical treatment	• Increased risk of adverse events • Short-term benefits • Continued low self-efficacy	• Self-management skills training • Interdisciplinary treatment programs

Adapted from reference 18.

guy," these assessments are designed to help formulate a treatment plan that maximizes the chance for successful treatment, minimizes adverse events, and provides a measure of confidence in the clinician's ability to properly manage the patient. For example, in our outpatient private practice clinic setting (authors LC and DMD), on any given day the staff pain psychologists are involved in risk assessment, evaluations for an opioid use disorder, discussions of opioid compliance and suggestions for revised compliance monitoring programs, spinal cord stimulator or neuromodulation evaluations, other presurgical evaluations, management of intrathecal pumps, brief behavioral interventions for insomnia/weight management/smoking cessation, coping skills training, biofeedback, mindfulness training, and individual therapy for grief/anxiety/depression or other mood disorders. A major activity is educating patients regarding the complexity of pain, setting realistic expectations, and clarifying the role that patients themselves play in successful long-term management of their disease. The psychologists work collaboratively with medical providers and physical therapists in a multidisciplinary setting. We also provide these services to practitioners in the community who do not have psychological services at their disposal on site. Our collective experience of over 55 years has taught us some valuable lessons regarding effective and efficient communication and patient management tools.

How to Locate Pain Psychologists in Your Area

For the interested clinician, there are several ways to go about locating a pain psychologist in your area:

1. You can contact your state board of examiners in psychology for a list of local licensed therapists and their practice specialties.
2. You can contact the department of psychology at a local university that offers a doctoral degree in psychology to determine if they are aware of former students who are practicing in the field of pain psychology.
3. Several regional and national pain societies, such as the American Academy of Pain Medicine, maintain a member roster by discipline and region.

Efforts to expand the availability of psychological services to surrounding areas have included the development of telepsychology, which allows psychologists to provide services to patients in remote sites (e.g., rural primary care settings), thus saving patients the inconvenience and expense of traveling. This program also helps to address the apparent shortage of appropriately trained and experienced pain psychologists and is responsive to a recent "call to action" issued by the American Academy of Pain Medicine Psychology Task Force.[19]

Patient–Clinician Interactions

The standard-of-care approach to patient–clinician interactions has largely moved away from the traditional "medical model" characterized by a paternalistic approach in which patients are not a large part of the decision-making process. Some patients find it reassuring when the clinician assumes the role of authority; they may be confused about their symptoms, the meaning of these symptoms, what tests will be most revealing, and how to evaluate treatment options. However, others see this approach as condescending and dictatorial. They feel ignored and discounted, which in turn influences their compliance. The perception that the clinician does not listen or is being insensitive or disrespectful is a common reason patients leave their doctor. Feeling coerced and angry and believing that the doctor is financially motived are common reasons patients file lawsuits.[20,21] Conversely, trusting the doctor and feeling every effort was made to help, independent of the actual outcome, are protective factors. Developing and implementing effective communication skills can not only improve outcomes but also help to avoid embarrassing or litigious situations.

The tide in clinician–patient relationships has shifted to incorporate terminology such as *patient-centered, person-centered,* and *person-directed care* (Table 1.2 provides distinctions).[22] Any experienced clinician has encountered patients who demand certain tests and/or treatments. Those patients perceive the clinician's role as merely rubber-stamping their proposals. This is a common trait among educated younger generations who are comfortable in the driver's seat, but also in older generations who now have access to a myriad of information, both correct and incorrect, through the internet (aka "Dr. Google"). Although patient requests are sometimes accurate and warranted, self-diagnosis is frustrating, can increase somatic anxiety, and may lead to unnecessary tests and health care charges. Thus, providers understandably might be reluctant to swing to the other extreme of the continuum and relinquish control.

In *patient-centered care*, the patient is allowed to make an informed decision together with the clinician. Patient-centered practitioners respect and respond to the individual's "preferences, needs and values"[23] and employ a variety of therapeutic and communication skills.

Table 1.2 Types of clinician–patient relationship

Characteristics	Patient-Centered	Person-Centered	Person-Directed
Role of clinician in decision-making	Moderate	Moderate	Moderate
Role of patient in decision-making	Moderate	Moderate	High
Importance of nonmedical issues	Moderate	High	Very high
Empowerment/ education of patients/ support persons	Moderate	Moderate	Very high
Coordination of care	Low	Moderate	Very high

Adapted from reference 22.

Person-centered care has been used interchangeably with the preceding term but connotes a broader focus on the whole person, not just the patient's medical condition. This likely becomes more salient for people suffering from chronic diseases like chronic pain. In the case of chronic pain, a person-centered appointment could manifest in a discussion involving not just pain severity reduction, but also attention to mood, function, and improvement in overall quality of life. Patients are treated as active partners with their clinician, and providers appreciate patients not only from a clinical/medical perspective, but also from an emotional, mental, spiritual, cultural, and social perspective. A respectful, trusting relationship obviously improves this partnership and the patient's willingness to listen to medical evidence and expertise. Patients may relinquish their participation in some circumstances, yielding to the clinician's recommendations. However, this is done only in the context of individually tailored information and documented informed consent. Conversely, clinicians may encourage patient autonomy, choice, and self-management in various aspects of lifestyle change interventions.

There is a consensus about what constitutes best practice for physician communication in medical encounters. It includes the following:

1. Fostering the relationship
2. Gathering information
3. Providing information
4. Making decisions
5. Responding to emotions
6. Enabling disease- and treatment-related behavior.

Indeed, the recent report from the U.S. Health and Human Services Pain Management Best Practice Inter-Agency Task Force notes, "A collaborative patient-clinician alliance, the cornerstone of best practices, has been eroded in our health care system. Reforms are needed to reduce administrative burden, increase face-to-face time with patients, and restore the patient-clinician relationship."[24]

Clinicians practicing person-centered care can improve their patients' clinical outcomes and satisfaction rates by improving the quality of the clinician–patient relationship. The person-centered encounter can involve any one or more of several goals, such as easing an emotionally distraught patient, providing education and clarification, and initiating behavioral change. Done properly, this approach has also proved effective at decreasing the use of diagnostic testing, prescriptions, hospitalizations, and referrals.[25]

Incorporating Psychological Techniques in Clinical Practice

In clinical practice, a premium is placed on efficiency and economy of effort as each encounter may last only a few minutes. The Socratic method of engaging the patient in critical thinking and decision-making (e.g., "Have you considered some ways that might work for you to quit smoking?") is often more palatable and productive than a more autocratic or dictatorial lecture ("You should quit smoking because I say so"). However, clinicians often worry that allowing the patient to open-endedly divulge information will consume precious time and potentially cloud the diagnostic picture with seemingly irrelevant complaints. An interesting study using audiotapes of primary care physician visits[26] suggested that in 25% of visits, the physician never asked for the patient's concerns at all. Patients making an initial problem statement were interrupted by their physician after an average of 23.1 seconds. However, patients who were allowed to complete their statement of concerns used only 6 seconds more on average than those who were redirected. So, with just a few extra seconds of patience and active listening, a clinician can let patients explore their own narrative and gather a story richer in symptom detail, psychosocial history, and context.

For example, consider a recent interaction one of us (LC) had with an interventional anesthesiologist during consultation for a cervical epidural block. Rather than saying, "I'm not sure this block will help, but we might as well try it anyway," the physician stated, "This block is designed to help reduce the inflammation around that disc and nerve. It has the best chance of helping if combined with your exercise program and stretching." In a matter of only seconds, the clinician provided education and realistic expectations with an optimistic slant and emphasized the importance of the patient's involvement in her own healing.

Likewise, in the process of assessing patients complaining of low back pain we often hear, "The doctor told me my back is *so bad* [or ... it's like a 90-year-old's, or ... I don't know how you're even walking!] *that even surgery will not help.*" This confers a sense of hopelessness on the patient and can leave the clinician stymied. The patient assumes the worst-case scenario and may now believe they are entitled to whatever it takes for them to be comfortable; treatment becomes a means of palliation rather than functional restoration. A pain psychologist can endeavor to help the patient correct this misperception. However, medical practitioners, especially the orthopedist or neurosurgeon in this case, tend to convey greater authority in medical matters. In this example, a more constructive conversation on the surgeon's part might have been, "You have several areas in your spine contributing to your pain. The outcome from any surgery would be very uncertain. The best chance for improvement is to be involved in a more comprehensive treatment program. This is likely to require participation on your part. But, at this time, it is the best approach." Such attention to communication, even in such brief interactions, can set up potent self-fulfilling prophecies.

Summary

Your interactions with patients with chronic pain can substantially influence patient compliance, treatment outcome, patient satisfaction, and your own level of stress. The meaning and context given to facts, as well as the empathy and consideration given to how the facts are delivered, may be more important than the facts themselves. In other words, how something is said can be more influential than what is actually said. This realization is well understood within placebo effect research, in which even analgesic responses can be initiated and maintained by patient expectations in the absence of an actual physiological intervention. Patient responses to contextual factors—such as clinician–patient communication styles—are not simply response biases but have clear neurobiological underpinnings.[27]

In a climate of increasing medical specialization, economic demands, and advanced technology, it is easy to lose sight of the human aspects involved in clinical practice. We encourage clinicians to find the most effective balance between the application of scientific algorithms and the art of clinical practice. Most clinicians will easily recognize the evidence-based principles and communication suggestions presented in this book. Our goal is to expand, refine, and simplify the application of these principles. Not every interaction will unfold as you would wish, but there are ways to approach patient encounters that can leave you feeling more confident in your attempts. The case scenarios we present have been extrapolated from our own experience and those most commonly brought to our attention by other clinicians and medical providers. In this regard, we hope to replicate real-life encounters versus presenting hypothetical situations. We are optimistic that the guidelines and techniques we present can help you feel more in control of and satisfied with your professional life and enhance the overall atmosphere of your practice.

References

1. McCue JD. The effects of stress on physicians and their medical practice. *N Engl J Med* 1982;306:458–463.
2. Alan HR. The impact of stress, burnout, and personality on physician attitudes and behaviors that impact patient care. *Psychol Behav Sci Int J* 2017;3(1):1–3.
3. O'Dowd TC. Five years of heartsink patients in general practice. *BMJ* 1988;297:528–530.
4. St. Sauver J, Warner DO, Yawn BP, Jacobson DJ, McGree ME, Pankratz JJ, Melton LJ III, Roger VL, Ebbert JO, Rocca WA. Why do patients visit their doctors? Assessing the most prevalent conditions in a defined US population. *Mayo Clin Proc* 2013;88(1):56–67.
5. International Association for the Study of Pain. Pain terms: a list with definitions and notes on usage. *Pain* 1979;6:249–252.
6. Siddall PJ, Cousins MJ. Persistent pain as a disease entity: implications for clinical management. *Anesth Analg* 2004;99:510–520.
7. Price TJ, Gold MS. From mechanism to cure: renewing the goal to eliminate the disease of pain. *Pain Med* 2018;19(8):1525–1549.
8. Borsook D, Becerra L, Hargraves R. Biomarkers for chronic pain and analgesia. Part 1: The need, reality, challenges, and solutions. *Discov Med* 2011;11(58):197–207.
9. Niculescu AB, Le-Niculescu H, Levey DE, Roseberry K, Soe KC, Rogers J, Khan F, Jones T, Judd S, McCormick MA, Wessel AR, Williams A, Kurian SM, White FA. Towards precision medicine for pain: diagnostic biomarkers and repurposed drugs. *Mol Psychiatry* 2019;24:501–522.
10. Scott-Warren J. Book review: "Pain Comorbidities: Understanding and Treating the Complex Patient," M. A. Giamberardino and T. S. Jensen (editors). *Br J Anaesth* 2014;113(5):888.

11. Bair MJ, Robinson RL, Katon W, Kroenke K. Depression and pain comorbidity: a literature review. *JAMA Intern Med* 2003;163(20):2433–2445.

12. Barry DT, Irwin KS, Jones ES, Becker WC, Tetrault JM, Sullivan LE, Hansen H, O'Connor PG, Schottenfeld RS, Fiellin DA. Opioids, chronic pain, and addiction in primary care. *J Pain* 2010;11(12):1442–1450.

13. Hurter S, Palovelis Y, Williams, AC, Fotopouou A. Partners' empathy increases pain ratings: effects of perceived empathy and attachment style on pain report and display. *J Pain* 2014;15(9):934–944.

14. Tang NK, Salkovskis PM, Hodges A, Wright KJ, Hanna M, Hester J. Effects of mood on pain responses and pain tolerance: an experimental study in chronic back pain patients. *J Pain* 2008;138(2):392–401.

15. Levine FM, DeSimone LL. The effects of experimenter gender on pain report in male and female subjects. *Pain* 1991;44(1):69–72.

16. Flor H, Kerns RD, Turk DC. The role of spouse reinforcement, perceived pain, and activity levels of chronic pain patients. *J Psychosom Res* 1987;31:251–259.

17. Lee H, McAuley JH, Hübscher M, Kamper SJ, Traeger AC, Moseley GL. Does changing pain-related knowledge reduce pain and improve function through changes in catastrophizing? *Pain* 2016;157:922–930.

18. Linton SJ, Shaw WS. Impact of psychological factors in the experience of pain. *Phys Ther* 2011;91(5): 700–711.

19. Darnall BD, Scheman J, Davin S, Burns JW, Murphy JL, Wilson AC, Kerns RD, Mackey SC. Pain psychology: a global needs assessment and national call to action. *Pain Med* 2016;17(2):250–263.

20. Vincent C, Young M, Phillips A. Why do people sue doctors? A study of patients and relatives taking legal action. *Lancet* 1994;343(8913):1609–1613.

21. Fishbain DA, Bruns D, Disorbio JM, Lewis JE. What are the variables that are associated with the patient's wish to sue his physician in patients with acute and chronic pain? *Pain Med* 2008;9:1130–1142.

22. Kumar R, Chattu VK. What is in the name? Understanding terminologies of patient-centered, person-centered, and patient-directed care. *J Family Med Prim Care* 2018;7(3):487–488.

23. Institute of Medicine Committee on Quality of Health Care in America;. *Crossing the Quality Chasm: A New Health System for the 21st Century.* Washington, DC: IOM, 2001.

24. Cheng J, Rutherford M, Singh VM. The HHS Pain Management Inter-Agency Best Practice Task Force Report calls for patient-centered and individualized care. *Pain Med* 2020;21(1):1–3; quotation is on p. 2.

25. King A, Hoppe RB. "Best practice" for patient-centered communication: a narrative review. *J Grad Med Educ* 2013;5(3):385–393.

26. Marvel MK, Epstein RM, Flower K, Beckman HB. Soliciting the patient's agenda: have we improved? *JAMA* 1999;281(3):283–287.

27. Price DD, Finniss DG, Benedetti F. A comprehensive review of the placebo effect: recent advance and current thought. *Annu Rev Psychol* 2008;59:565–590.

Further Reading

ACOG Committee Opinion 587. Effective physician-patient communication. *Obstet Gynecol* 2014;123(2):389–393.

Cianfrini LR, Block C, Doleys DM. Psychological therapies. In Deer TR (editor-in-chief), *Comprehensive Treatment of Chronic Pain by Medical, Interventional, and Integrative Approaches: The American Academy of Pain Management Textbook on Patient Management.* New York: Springer, 2013:827–844.

Cianfrini LR, Doleys DM. The role of psychology in pain management. *Pract Pain Manag* 2006;6:18–28.

Darnell B. *Psychological Treatment for Patients with Chronic Pain.* Washington, DC: American Psychological Association Press, 2018.

Doleys DM. *Understanding and Managing Chronic Pain: A Guide for the Patient and Clinician.* Denver, CO: Outskirts Press, 2014.

Doleys DM, Cianfrini LR. Psychological assessment and neuromodulation for pain. In Turk D, Gatchel R (eds.), *Psychological Approaches to Pain Management.* 3rd ed. New York: Guilford, 2018:303–318.

Newton BW. Walking a fine line: is it possible to remain an empathic physician and have a hardened heart. *Front Hum Neurosci* 2013;7(233):1–13.

Travado L, Grassi L, Gil F, Ventura C, Martins C. Southern European Psycho-Oncology Study Group. Physician-patient communication among southern European cancer physicians: the influence of psychosocial orientation and burnout. *Psychooncology* 2005;14(8):661–670.

U.S. Department of Health and Human Services Pain Management Best Practices Inter-Agency Task Force. *Pain Management Best Practices Inter-Agency Task Force Report: Updates, Gaps, Inconsistencies, and Recommendations. Final Report.* Washington, DC: HHS, 2019. https://www.hhs.gov/ash/advisory-committees/pain/reports/index.html

2

Core Communication Skills in Health Care

Elizabeth J. Richardson

Case: "A Refill on Drugs" or "a Medication Refill:" The Power of Words

Suppose you're getting ready to see your last two patients for the day. You open their charts to read initial notes from staff before entering the room. In Chart 1, you read, "Patient is here to get a refill on his drugs." In Chart 2, you read, "Patient is here for a routine medication refill." We could even go further: the patient in Chart 1 "hasn't been complying with your recommendations" and the patient in Chart 2 "has been non-adherent to exercise recommendations." We have all read "Chart 1" notes and experienced dread about opening the clinic door to begin the assessment, expecting hostility at worst and polite refusal to follow recommendations at best. Indeed, primary care physicians describe working with patients to manage their chronic pain as frustrating and often stressful.[1] The encouraging news is that such negative experiences can be lessened or even avoided by enhancing your communication skills.[1]

Challenge: How to Recognize Biases That Impede Effective Communication

Communication is more than a simple verbal exchange between two parties. For communication to be truly effective, we must understand both our own mental framework and that of the other person with whom we are communicating. One of the remarkable feats of the human brain is higher-order cognition—that is, the ability to reason, plan, solve complex problems, and make decisions. Moreover, we can do this in a very efficient manner, using cognitive processes that take in new information and organize it based on what we've already experienced.[2] The reality is, however, that this ability can come at a cost: we are often less-than-rational thinkers in our daily routines. If we were to rationally and systematically examine all possible outcomes of every decision or response we make, we would never get through the day! A routine grocery run could take hours if we weighed and deliberated each possible aspect of choosing one apple over another. Color, texture, sheen, cost, size, location in the bin—your brain takes in mounds of data. If you are like most people, you tend to make such everyday decisions automatically, without much conscious effort,[2] to the tune of "what feels right." In other words, we rely in our thinking on mental shortcuts or *heuristics*, of which we are not necessarily conscious.

We base mental heuristics partially on situational context. For example, let's suppose that you and your spouse are about to leave to go out to dinner at a restaurant. Your spouse asks, "Are you ready?" Your tone and response may likely be completely different than your response to the waiter at the restaurant who asks the very same question. The use of a heuristic in this case, based on the situational context, allowed you to select an appropriate answer without laboriously going through all possible answers to that particular question.

Similarly, the way in which information is framed can also affect our appraisal of a situation, the characteristics of an object or individual that we perceive, and ultimately the decisions we make within that context. People will consistently rate ground beef as better when it is labeled "75% lean" rather than "25% fat," even though it's the same thing.[3] When evaluating a proposed treatment that would save 72% of lives versus that which would allow 28% to die, the former is rated as more appealing even though it's an equivalent expected value.[4] The effect of framing has also been shown to affect clinicians' perceptions and their approach to managing pain. In one study,[5] providers were given chart notes that contained either objectively phrased descriptions of the patient or descriptions that contained subtle bias. Biased wording included the use of quotation marks (e.g., pain is "still a 10"), implying doubt of the patient, or other phrases that shift blame to the patient (e.g., "he refuses recommendations" vs. "he is not tolerating"). When chart information contained the biased wording, providers were less aggressive in their approach to managing patients' pain.[5] Put simply, any differences in the emotional reaction you experienced in reading our two example "charts" at the beginning of this chapter was likely due to how their information was framed to you, even though the patients' reasons for their visit were virtually the same.

When learning effective communication skills in the health care setting, understanding the dynamic nature of clinician–patient communication is crucial. While you have the expertise to assist patients with their problems, at the most basic level, you both are human and thus both bring previously learned beliefs, biases, and mental heuristics to the line of communication.

Clinician Context: Improving Awareness of Clinician Biases and Employing Empathy Can Improve the Therapeutic Alliance with the Patient

The patient and the clinician are not equal in their therapeutic relationship. Consoli and Consoli[6] outline the reasons for this nicely, and we can put their rationale into the context of pain management. A patient comes to you because they want relief from their pain, and you possess the necessary expertise to help solve their problem. In turn, you may have your own expectations of the relationship. The patient may unrealistically anticipate a "cure," and perhaps you overestimate their level of compliance and positive outcome. In either or both cases, the stage is set for the mismatch between our expectation and what actually develops within the relationship. One problem is that social interactions do not occur within a vacuum, guided by only the context or moment at hand. Not only are we affected by the language used in that interaction, but the social exchange is also shaped by preconceptions formed from past social interactions. In other words, a patient may unconsciously *transfer* feelings, beliefs, or assumptions learned in prior social encounters onto you, the clinician. However, this tendency is not unidirectional: the clinician also has a rich history of social encounters and may experience a *countertransference* of emotions in response to the patient's transference. While the terms *transference* and *countertransference* were born out of traditional Freudian views,[7] they offer a helpful framework within which to characterize the mental heuristics we use to quickly assess the motives of an individual and our responses—at times to the detriment of the patient–clinician working relationship.

Examples of transference, countertransference, and potential problems within the provider–patient relationship in pain management

Transference	Countertransference	Potential Problem
Placing unrealistic expectations on the clinician **Example:** "Doc, you have got to fix this!"	Clinicians may feel they are put in an impossible situation, feelings of failure to help	Attempts to appease; reinforce passive management of pain and reliance on others to manage their pain
Relating the clinician to someone in their personal life **Example:** "Doctor, you remind me of my daughter. She is smart, kind, and would do anything to help people."	Positive feelings about this idealization; feeling a special bond with this particular patient	Responding as a friend rather than as a professional with focus on self-management of pain
Projecting past negative relationship experiences on the clinician **Example:** "You are like every everybody else I've seen. Taking away medications when people like me need them most!"	Recalling past patients' manipulative and/or drug-seeking behaviors; feeling anger toward the patient	Avoidance, bias in prescriptive recommendations "to teach" or attempt to control patient behavior

Countertransference highlights the importance of examining our own motives and biases, and not just those of the patient. When you open the door to the clinic room to evaluate the patient, what is your emotional reaction? Does this patient remind you of a fond loved one? Have you had personal experience with a loved one with addiction or chronic health condition, and are you finding yourself wanting to respond in similar ways as you did with that loved one? You cannot erase all of your personal experiences—nor should you—but you can become mindful of the effect your experiences have on the patient–clinician relationship.

When addressing transference and countertransference issues, the goal is not to be devoid of emotion or to become stilted in your responses to patients. We are humans, not automatons. Rather, use those feelings when you detect them as a barometer of the psychosocial factors the patient may be bringing to the table. Perhaps the demanding patient is coming from a place of anxiety and catastrophic thinking. Perhaps the patient who projects a previous close relationship is lacking in social support. Perhaps if you could "peel back" the anger from the accusatory patient, might you see a fear of unmanageability of their pain? Using these as "measures" in your assessment can ultimately improve the patient–clinician relationship and can alert you to other domains that may be contributing to the patient's pain experience.

In psychotherapy, the quality of the relationship between the clinician and the patient—the *therapeutic alliance*—consistently contributes to patient outcomes, irrespective of treatment modality.[8,9] In short, a stronger alliance between patient and clinician appears to be foundational in achieving positive outcomes. Bordin[10] outlined the important ingredients of an effective alliance: (1) mutually agreed-upon *goals*, or outcomes, (2) mutually agreed-upon *tasks*, or strategies used to reach those goals, and (3) an emotional connection or *bond* consisting of trust, acceptance, and confidence within the relationship. The question is, then, what facilitates a good working relationship or alliance? Prior research emphasizes that a clinician's empathic communication is the catalyst. Specifically, the level of provider empathy positively influences the degree of alliance, which in turn promotes more positive outcomes for the patient.[11,12] McClintock and others[11] found that the patient–clinician agreement on the goals and tasks (components of alliance) are most positively influenced by empathy. In our experience, facilitating agreement involves finding common ground, which can be inherent in empathic communication. Most often, this includes stating larger, obvious goals (e.g., "getting pain to a manageable level" or "reducing how much pain interferes with activities") versus more clinically oriented goals that are often jargon-laden and difficult for the patient to interpret (e.g., "ambulating 200 feet without an assistive device" or "increasing range of motion").

"Empathy or Sympathy? I'm Confused"

As humans, there are a multitude of emotions we can experience when encountering someone in need and, more specifically, in pain. Sadness, frustration, sympathy, irritation—the emotions are complex and diverse. The words *sympathy* and *empathy* are often used synonymously, but actually they differ with respect to the frame of mind of the one expressing it.[6] Sympathy involves feeling *for* the other person, such as feeling pity about their plight. Empathy involves feeling *with* the other person and shifting your thoughts to contemplate the other person's point of view.[13] Sympathy involves somewhat of an emotionally distant observation of another person, whereas empathy involves mentally placing yourself "in their shoes" to understand the root of their emotional expression occurring in the present moment. In the bustle of a busy clinic day, our minds are continuously in "conceptualization mode," analyzing the patient's past history of symptoms while navigating a decision tree of future treatment. Paradoxically, empathic communication requires self-awareness of your own emotions in the moment,[14] thus making it a very mindful approach. In this way, empathy provides a mechanism by which the clinician can "accept the patient's doubts and fears, and their moments of despondency or rebellion, without interpreting them as a lack of confidence in them or as a criticism of their therapeutic suggestions" (p. 19).[6]

How do we engage in empathy? Wiseman[13] outlined four defining attributes of empathic communication:

1. Seeing the world as your patient sees it
2. Maintaining objectivity and a nonjudgmental stance (e.g., acknowledging your own biases and heuristics, with an attempt to defuse them)
3. Understanding the other person's feelings
4. Communicating that understanding to the other individual.

Let's see this at work.

A patient who is undergoing an opioid taper is angry and states, "Pain has ruined my life, and now you are going to take away the only thing that has helped me!" Understandably, as the clinician, my initial emotional reaction to this patient's statement may be frustration and defensiveness. However, I can choose to observe my reaction without reacting to it (maintaining objectivity). In an attempt to shift to my patient's point of view, I may recognize that he is likely perceiving manageability of his pain as outside of his control (seeing the world as he sees it) and that he is attempting to control the only way he knows how (understanding his feelings). This would particularly be true if medication was the only method of pain management the patient had experienced to that point and he had not been provided education surrounding the complexity of factors contributing to the pain experience. Instead of leaping into a recitation of what may be certainly valid, scientific reasons for the medication taper, which could strain the therapeutic alliance, I would be best served to initially reflect back my understanding of that patient's emotions. For example: "Your pain has certainly affected every facet of your life. I would be angry too if I thought there was only one way to manage my pain and it would no longer be available." This not only communicates understanding of the patient's feelings but also provides an opening to discussing the development of self-management strategies and the importance of pain psychology. Indeed, when clinicians are perceived as nonjudgmental, supportive, and understanding of patients' fears, patients are more amenable to non-opioid pain management strategies and tapering.[15,16]

It is important to emphasize that taking a step back to observe our own emotion is not the same as restricting or overly regulating our emotion. Empathic communication is not only what is said and how we say it, but also our accompanying nonverbal cues, such as emotional expression. Particularly in professional contexts, we may become emotionally detached when faced with tense patient interactions under the false assumption that such detachment maintains objectivity.[17,18] However, emotional distancing, rather than acknowledging, appears to place greater strain on the patient–clinician relationship in such situations.[19] Emotionally detaching or distancing in tense interactions not only will limit your ability to recognize and reflect on your own emotions (e.g., countertransference), but it may also impede your ability to garner clues about the patient's underlying emotions (e.g., using countertransference as a gauge).[17]

Patient Context: A Patient's Thoughts, Expectations, and Sense of Self-Agency Predict Outcomes and Can Be Influenced in Communication with the Clinician

We now know that the experience of pain is not simply a function of nociceptive input. Rather, pain is a complex interplay of social, psychological, cognitive, and biological factors, which has given rise to understanding pain from the biopsychosocial model. Still, we sometimes silo these constructs during treatment without realizing their truly interactive nature. Thought processes and language—from within our social sphere to our own self-talk—can have an impact not only on patient emotions but also the degree of pain experienced.

The Power of Thought

Henry Beecher was one of the first to note that expectations about the meaning and course of pain impact the pain we experience. In his work, he found that soldiers wounded in battle and treated at field hospitals required less pain medication than civilians with similar injuries.[20] His interpretation was that the pain had disparate meanings to those two groups: either marking the beginning of tragedy and loss of the life the patient knew, or the end of tragedy by being removed from the battlefield due to the injury. Similarly, those who held more positive expectations about recovery acutely following injuries actually fared better physically when reassessed at later time points.[21] One well-known example of how outcomes can be impacted by expectations (which in turn can be shaped by what we are told and how we interpret cues) is the placebo effect.

The Inseparable Mind and Body: The Benefits of Placebo

In medicine, the placebo is considered fundamental to clinical trials. If a clinical trial shows a treatment to have no benefit over placebo, then it is deemed non-efficacious. Yet, the placebo itself has been shown to offer relief in pain.[22,23] Given recent and mounting problems with the use of opioids to manage chronic pain, there has been renewed interest in better understanding the psychological factors contributing to placebo analgesia. For example, is the driving factor what the patient is told, the nonverbal cues associated with taking "a pill," or the manner in which the provider interacts with that individual?

There is evidence that placebo, an inert substance, can directly affect the body's own pain-reducing mechanisms. Levine, Gordon, and Fields[23] gave dental patients either morphine or saline following oral surgery, with those receiving saline also exhibiting pain relief. Interestingly, however, when patients who received saline were also given naloxone, an opioid receptor antagonist, the placebo response disappeared. This, among other work,[24] suggests that simply the belief in or expectation for relief is powerful enough to influence our own endogenous opioid system in positive ways.

Most have assumed that deception is necessary to establish patients' expectations in order to obtain relief from placebo, yet this is not the case. Surprisingly, individuals still experience placebo relief from pain when they are informed that they are taking inert substances. Individuals with chronic low back pain still experienced significantly greater pain reduction during their usual care when given a placebo and told about it.[25] Among those with chronic recurrent migraines, open-label placebo was associated with significantly improved pain compared to no treatment.[26] At least neurologically, the brain appears to react to contextual cues outside of conscious awareness that contribute to the placebo effect.[27]

What are potential contextual cues? Some cues may be differences in phrasing and body language of the person communicating to the patient. In one study,[28] the degree of spinal compression and lumbar muscle tension was recorded as individuals without pain performed a lifting task. Unbeknownst to the participants, they had actually been randomized into one of two conditions. In one condition, the examiner smiled, nodded, established good eye contact, and provided frequent encouragement. In the other condition, the examiner behaved in a somewhat opposite manner: little eye contact, no supportive language, and a focus on what the participant was doing incorrectly. The researchers found that participants in the latter condition with negative contextual cues exhibited greater lumbar disc compression and muscle tension.[28]

There is also evidence that empathic communication affects the placebo response. Fuentes and others[29] assigned individuals with chronic low back pain to receive either active or sham (placebo) electrotherapy by a provider who communicated empathically versus one with limited interaction during the therapy session. In the empathic communication condition, patients were asked about their symptoms and providers often summarized what patients said to demonstrate understanding. Providers in the empathy group also engaged in nonverbal behaviors, such as maintaining eye contact with the patient. While the active plus empathic communication group showed the most benefit, patients still experienced significantly reduced pain in the sham condition as long as the provider communicated empathically.[29] Likewise, when patients were not only asked about their symptoms but were also asked in a manner that demonstrated "being heard" (e.g., the provider asking questions back to clarify the patient's responses), patients experienced significantly more symptom relief and improvements in quality of life during sham acupuncture.[30] Patients also experienced greater relief when the clinician asked more comprehensive questions about emotional, psychological, and other broad domains of functioning rather than narrowly focusing questions on symptom history.[31]

Self-Efficacy

In other medical conditions, such as diabetes, empathy from the clinician is associated with improved beliefs on the part of patients about their own ability to effectively cope with their symptoms.[32] This belief in our ability to exert positive change may underlie why we see the effect of clinician empathy on more concrete clinical outcomes, such as improved hemoglobin A1c levels[33] and reduced duration of the common cold.[34]

In a large survey of individuals with chronic pain,[35] those who perceived their medical team as empathic and collaborative had higher *self-efficacy*, or the belief in their ability to effect change in their situation. This, in turn, was related to less pain intensity and pain interference.

The terms *self-esteem* and *self-efficacy* are often confused. While self-esteem involves a more global evaluation about ourselves, self-efficacy refers more to our sense of agency. Specifically, self-efficacy refers to our belief in our ability to exert influence on events or situations through our own behavior.[36] Bandura[36] outlined four ways in which self-efficacy can be increased:

1. Facing a task or challenge and experiencing mastery of it. In short, prior successes give us confidence that we can succeed again when encountering additional challenges.

2. Social modeling. When we see others effect change in a certain situation, it can boost our confidence that we can also have an impact.
3. Social persuasion. We may not initially feel that we have the ability to manage aspects of our life, but we can be convinced that we do indeed have that capability. This is similar to the power of belief and expectation we see from placebo research. Likewise, it is not necessary to mislead or deceive patients by falsely inflating their capabilities, nor should that be what we attempt with social persuasion. Rather, it is important to highlight the very real benefits of patients' use of self-management strategies for chronic pain.
4. Changing our current mood state. It likely does not come as a surprise that when we are in a good mood, we tend to be more confident in our abilities. If depressed or stressed, we become less confident.

Developing Self-Efficacy for the Patient with Chronic Pain

Self-Efficacy Source	Ways to Develop	What to Avoid
Personal Mastery	Setting small, specific, and achievable goals that are measurable in terms of self-improvement. **Examples:** "How about we make a goal of walking to your mailbox to retrieve the mail each afternoon?" or "Let's increase your daily walking by 5 minutes."	Creating large, vague goals that can set the person up to fail. Comparing success/failure to the progress of others. **Examples:** "We need to increase your activity levels" or "Adding a walking program to your daily routine will help with your pain."
Social Modeling	Seeing others effectively manage their pain, or if this is not possible, describing your experiences with patients who have experienced success. **Example:** "I have had patients who were in your situation with back pain, and they are now managing their pain instead of having their pain manage them."	Lack of examples, either first-hand or relayed through your conversations with the patient

Self-Efficacy Source	Ways to Develop	What to Avoid
Social Persuasion	Emphasizing positive language when describing treatment options. There is a reason you are selecting certain options for the patient, and that is usually because they can offer benefit. Highlight those benefits. **Examples:** "These are strategies you can implement at any stage of the game" or "I feel confident these are ways we can manage your pain."	Using negative or neutral language that may highlight unfavorable outcomes. **Example:** "People may experience different results with these treatments," "Depending on the person, the treatment may or may not work," or "Self-management is difficult for a lot of people to accept, but ..."
Mood State	Helping patients to reinterpret negative bias and rely less on their physical state to guide their behavior. Examples: "Pain does not always mean harm is happening to your body, though our emotions may tell us otherwise" or "Some activities in the past may have hurt, but what activities—no matter how small—have you been able to do?"	Working around a patient's emotional or physical state. "When you feel rested, let's try walking around the block" or "On a day you feel more upbeat, make a plan to go the gym."

Adapted from Bandura's (1994) four sources of self-efficacy.

In essence, a provider's words can be quite powerful in building patients' self-efficacy to implement effective emotional and behavioral coping strategies to best manage their pain. When providers were trained to convey positive expectations versus making cautious or provisional statements, it was predictive of the patient's self-efficacy three months later.[37] Further, higher patient self-efficacy in turn predicts lower pain levels.[37]

Communication: Use of Certain Communication Strategies Can Foster Self-Efficacy, Overcome Resistance, and Close the Divide Between Patient Behaviors and Functional Goals

In chronic conditions, the focus is often on implementing long-term solutions to help patients best manage their symptoms to live life more fully. Herein lies a problem: clinicians cannot do this for patients. Patients must assume ownership of necessary self-management tools to improve their lives outside of your office. Yet, how many times have you made recommendations—whether it is to see a pain psychologist or to increase exercise—only to find during subsequent visits that your patient did not follow through?

As the clinician, you have the knowledge about what would best help the patient. You present facts and figures, and give empirically supported advice on what behaviors will better manage their symptoms. As an expert, you may tend to have a "righting reflex"[38] and make the case as to why patients should do this or that, or why what they are doing is not helping them or is even hurting them. This "directing" communication style is common among health care providers;[38] after all, you *do* know the solution to their problem. However, what typically comes next highlights a common paradox in patient–clinician relationships: the more we advise, tell, or teach, the greater the tendency for the patient to counter. For example, instructing patients to reduce their alcohol intake may be met with "It's not really a problem" or "It's not like *that*, doc—I can quit anytime."

Motivational interviewing (MI) is a communication strategy adopted by clinicians to avoid this impasse. MI, when implemented well, can help the patient shift toward adopting positive health behaviors and therefore attain better clinical outcomes. While it was first used with individuals battling alcohol use disorders,[39] MI has since been applied by clinicians to help patients implement change toward symptom improvement across a number of chronic health conditions.[38,40] Among older adults with chronic pain, use of MI was associated with increased self-efficacy and decreased risk of opioid misuse.[41] When MI strategies were paired with conventional physical therapy for chronic low back pain, patients perceived their general health as better and exhibited greater compliance with exercise programs.[42] One systematic review of MI in chronic pain showed only small to moderate effects with respect to patient compliance, and outcomes in physical functioning were questionable.[43] However, this does not necessarily imply that use of MI strategies does not produce clinical returns; rather, MI methods may be *one* important component in the trajectory of progress. In a path analysis, Cheing and others[44] found that MI strategies improved the therapeutic alliance, which in turn was related to patients expecting better outcomes from treatment. It was this last "domino" of patient expectation that influenced clinical outcomes of pain intensity and physical functioning.[44]

At the heart of MI is the notion that active listening can serve as fertile ground for the provider to elicit change within the patient. This is not to say that the clinician's knowledge and the conveying of that knowledge is not foundational in the relationship; in fact, that is why the patient seeks your care. Instead, MI is a strategic way of asking, listening, and informing in a manner that maximizes the patient's motivation and commitment to change.[38] In MI, there is more emphasis on understanding the patient's motivations and the fact that any areas of concern the patient identifies are likely the ripest for eliciting change.[38,45] This is because we all tend to have the greatest strife over decisions or behaviors about which we are ambivalent, and when there is ambivalence, there is opportunity to help the patient tip the balance toward positive behavioral change. One way to accomplish this is to highlight the discrepancy between the patient's current behaviors and the functional goals reported by the patient.[45]

Rollnick and colleagues[38] suggest that when meeting with a patient, it is helpful to set a collaborative agenda and allow the patient to choose a topic of concern. Providing a check sheet at the beginning of the visit can facilitate this process or be used to revisit areas as necessary.[38] As agenda items are successfully addressed, the check sheet can serve as a prompt to continue to prioritize and focus on areas of self-improvement. Further, patients can use a 0-to-10 numeric rating scale to assess how important it is for them to "move better," "engage in more activities," or make progress in whatever area they identify. This measurement can then be used to track change and review with the patient on subsequent visits.[38] At least when it concerns behavior change, it is our experience that it is more effective to focus on domains impacted by pain rather than the pain intensity itself.

Sample Priority Check Sheet for Patients with Chronic Pain

_____ Pain fluctuating too much in the day

_____ Completing important tasks

_____ Engaging in hobbies and/or social activities

_____ Sexual functioning

_____ Sleep

_____ Medicines

_____ Stress

_____ Getting moving

_____ Other:_____

Adapted from Rollnick et al. (2008) to reflect areas of concern frequently experienced by individuals with chronic pain

When eliciting information from a patient, using open-ended versus closed-ended questions can provide a better opportunity for you to identify areas of ambivalence. For example, asking "How has the walking plan been working out for you?" rather than "Are you walking like we talked about before?" allows patient to expand on concerns, fear of movement, low perceived self-efficacy, or other obstacles to aligning the patient's behaviors with functional goals. Without asking open-ended questions that elucidate reasons behind the ambivalence, we may tend to blame the patient as simply making no effort, and barriers to progress will endure.

In MI, listening is an active process because it requires you to resist the urge to "make your case" when encountering resistance from the patient. In addition, it requires avoiding reassurance-type language, which can be well intended but also dismissive. Phrases like "It will be fine" or "What you are afraid of is very unlikely to occur" are often said with the intent to mitigate a patient's distress. After all, clinicians are trained to heal and, when time is of utmost value at the clinic, it is certainly an efficient response. Yet, when we instead "roll with resistance" rather than debating the facts or offering reassurances, we paradoxically are more likely to influence change.[46] When the patient appears resistant, reflective listing—or summarizing back what you are hearing the patient tell you—can help the patient feel understood, highlight discrepancies between the patient's current behaviors and goals, and move the patient toward change.

Examples of Reflection, Rolling with Resistance, and Highlighting Discrepancies

Provider	"You mentioned that physical therapy would not work for you. Tell me more about that."	Reflecting the resistance, asking open-ended question
Patient	"Moving aggravates my pain. I just can't afford to make it worse."	
Provider	"So, you are concerned that they will have you doing more exercise, and that your pain will increase, making it harder to cope."	Rolling with resistance, reflecting
Patient	"Yes, taking care of my responsibilities and completing activities is already hard. I certainly don't want to do more damage than I've already done to my back."	
Provider	"You are afraid that moving more might harm you further, yet I'm also hearing that completing activities is very important to you. That must feel like a tough spot to be in."	Reflecting, setting up discrepancy, avoiding flooding patient with facts
Patient	"I just don't know how to not make this any worse, and the medications are the only things that keep the pain stable. I mean, how do people with back pain do that?"	
Provider	"Incorporating activity has been shown to be an important component to a pain management program, and we usually start really small—not like how you think of people who don't have pain working out at the gym. However, you are having a hard time seeing how this is possible."	Informing, but maintaining reflection of the patient's ambivalence
Patient	"I couldn't do aerobics or anything like I used to. What kind of exercise do you mean?"	
Provider	"You think of exercise as being high impact or lengthy. Often, it can be just starting with spending just a few minutes walking at your own pace. How do you feel about that?"	Informing, open-ended question to elicit other areas of concern
Patient	"Yeah, I don't think of exercise like that. That may be something I could try."	*Change talk*

Adapted from Rollnick et al. (2008) and revised to reflect potential areas of resistance individuals with chronic pain.

Psychotherapeutic Modalities in Chronic Pain: The Basics

MI is a *communication method* that can influence patients' intrinsic motivation for change; it should not be confused with psychotherapeutic modalities that focus on intervening with certain thoughts and behaviors.[47] However, as a clinician treating individuals with chronic pain, it is important to understand the basics of empirically supported psychotherapeutic strategies. Such knowledge can improve the quality of your referrals to trained pain psychologists and help you arm your patient with accurate information when you discuss such a referral. Further detail about such modalities and in-context case examples will be provided in other chapters of this book.

Cognitive–Behavioral Therapy (CBT) for Chronic Pain

CBT, which originated in the late 1970s from the work of psychiatrist Aaron Beck,[48] is based on the notion that our thoughts and appraisals of events and situations mediate the emotions we experience. This is similar to the mental *heuristics* or automatic patterns of thinking discussed earlier in this chapter. While they may not always lead to problems, automatic thoughts can exacerbate anxiety, depression, or poor coping with life stressors, such as living with chronic pain. For example, a patient who is experiencing a pain flare-up may interpret the increase in intensity as a sign of harm and, as a result, become more anxious. That individual may cope by avoiding activities, leading to disuse and deconditioning and therefore more pain, setting in place a cruel cycle. In such cases, automatic thoughts are considered maladaptive (i.e., creating distressing emotions and/or dysfunctional ways of coping). In the context of chronic pain, *catastrophizing* is a common automatic thought pattern that has been shown to be consistently predictive of clinical outcomes.[49] In CBT for chronic pain, the patient is taught strategies to identify, challenge, and replace catastrophic thought patterns or other cognitive distortions.[50,51] Often, the rationale is placed within gate control theory,[52] emphasizing the role of "top-down" factors, such as our thoughts, in opening or closing the gate on pain perception.[51] The behavioral components of CBT for chronic pain focus on helping the patient learn diaphragmatic breathing, progressive muscle relaxation, and time-based pacing to engage in activities without wide oscillations in pain, among other "tools" the patient can implement as self-management.[51,53] CBT for chronic pain is an efficacious treatment paradigm and has been on the front lines as a psychological intervention for many years.[54]

Acceptance and Commitment Therapy (ACT)

We opened this chapter by discussing unique human cognitive capabilities: abstract reasoning, planning, solving complex problems, and making sophisticated decisions. We interpret what we are currently experiencing by what we have learned from the past and what it may mean going forward. In other words, we spend a good bit of our mental lives analyzing the past and calculating the future. We infer meaning and a course of action simply from what our mind derives from a given context.[55,56] This process implies that while we may experience pain in the present moment, suffering is a conditioned negative internal experience to which we decide to respond.[56]

ACT, which was developed by Stephen Hayes,[56,57] is based on the notion that we can over-identify or become "fused" with our thoughts. As a result, thoughts can powerfully influence our actions. For example, if a person with chronic pain is asked to attend a social gathering, the *thought* of the social gathering may be enough to elicit pain-related anxiety, even though that person hasn't actually yet experienced the event. In turn, the person may avoid or decline the invitation, which then relieves the anxiety. Similar to MI, this highlights a behavioral discrepancy. Here, the person's behavior to control the anxiety from a preconceived idea has now placed them in opposition to what they truly value—being less limited by their pain and engaging in more activities.[56] In this way, acceptance means not acquiescing to the pain and suffering that our mental assessments create, but rather a willingness to re-engage in activities that work toward value-based goals despite those mental assessments.

In the example above, CBT would focus on changing the maladaptive thought or appraisal that the person holds about what will happen. In ACT, however, identifying such thoughts and restructuring them would be considered an attempt to control the thought, which can ultimately reinforce the "fusion" between a person's thoughts and their responses.[56] Instead, ACT helps the patient "defuse" or decouple from their thoughts, thereby reducing the influence thoughts have on emotional functioning and behavior. This is done through teaching mindfulness, a skill that allows us to simply notice our thoughts for what they are—just thoughts—without our responses being compelled by them.[58] There is mounting evidence that building the skill of mindfulness helps an individual cope more effectively with pain. When mindfulness is incorporated into chronic pain management, patients experience greater reductions in disability and affective components of pain when compared to usual care.[59] Interestingly, however, providing patients with CBT similarly produces better outcomes than just usual care.[59] Functional magnetic resonance imaging (fMRI) studies show that mindfulness may decrease connectivity between neural regions associated with affective and sensory-discriminative dimensions of pain[60] and may even work by increasing our endogenous opioid response to pain.[61]

In summary, provider communication involves more than simply the specific information conveyed to the patient. Effective communication starts with the understanding that communication is a dynamic process, with both the provider and the patient bringing past experiences, biases, and preconceived notions to the table. By increasing our awareness of these factors, we can modify or even use them to gauge the degree of alliance between parties and as an indicator of when to use effective communication strategies (e.g., "rolling with resistance") to restore any strains in the alliance and elicit positive change from the patient. Moreover, being equipped with information about available effective psychotherapies will aid in communicating with a patient at the time of such referral as well as deepen the provider's understanding of self-management strategies patients develop when involved in these treatments.

References

1. Matthias MS, Parpart AL, Nyland KA, Huffman MA, Stubbs DL, Sargent C, Bair MJ. The patient-provider relationship in chronic pain care: provider's perspectives. *Pain Med* 2010;11:1688–1697.

2. Kahnehan D. *Thinking, Fast and Slow*. New York: Farrar, Straus and Giroux, 2011.

3. Levin IP, Gaeth GJ. How consumers are affected by the framing of attribute information before and after consuming the product. *J Consumer Res* 1988;15:374–378.

4. Tversky A, Kahneman D. The framing of decisions and the psychology of choice. *Science* 1981;211:453–458.

5. Goddu AP, O'Conor KJ, Lanzkron S, Saheed MO, Saha S, Peek ME, Haywood C, Beach MC. Do words matter? Stigmatizing language and the transmission of bias in the medical record. *J Gen Intern Med* 2018;33(5):685–691.

6. Consoli SG, Consoli SM. Countertransference in dermatology. *Acta Derm Venerol* 2016;Suppl 217:18–21.

7. Freud S. *Dora: An Analysis of a Case of Hysteria.* New York: Simon & Schuster, 1963.

8. Horvath AO, Symonds BD. Relation between working alliance and outcome in psychotherapy: a meta-analysis. *J Couns Psychol* 1991;38:139–149.

9. Martin DJ, Garske JP, Davis MK. Relation of the therapeutic alliance with outcome and other variables: a meta-analytic review. *J Consult Clin Psychol* 2000;68:438–450.

10. Bordin ES. The generalizability of the psychoanalytic concept of the working alliance. *Psychotherapy Theory Res Practice* 1979;16:252–260.

11. McClintock AS, Anderson TM, Patterson CL, Wing EH. Early psychotherapeutic empathy, alliance, and client outcome: preliminary evidence of indirect effects. *J Clin Psychol* 2018;74:839–848.

12. Malin AJ, Pos AE. The impact of early empathy on alliance building, emotional processing, and outcome during experiential treatment of depression. *Psychother Res* 2015;25: 445–459.

13. Wiseman T. A concept analysis of empathy. *J Adv Nurs* 1996;23:1162–1167.

14. Burnard P. Sharing a viewpoint. *Senior Nurse* 1987;7(3):38–39.

15. Frank JW, Levy C, Matlock DD, Calcaterra SL, Mueller SR, Koester S, Binswanger IA. Patients' perspectives on tapering of chronic opioid therapy: a qualitative study. *Pain Med* 2016;17:1838–1847.

16. Matthias MS, Johnson NL, Shields CG, Bair MJ, MacKie P, Huffman M, Alexander SC. "I'm not going to pull the rug out from under you": patient-provider communication about opioid tapering. *J Pain* 2017;18(11):1365–1373.

17. Halpern J. Empathy and patient-physician conflicts. *J Gen Intern Med* 2007;22(5):696–700.

18. Roter DL, Stewart M, Putnam SM, Lipkin M Jr, Stiles W, Inui TS. Communication patterns of primary care physicians. *JAMA* 1997;277(4):350–356.

19. Yagil D, Shnapper-Cohen M. When authenticity matters most: physician's regulation of emotional display and patient satisfaction. *Patient Educ Couns* 2016;99:1694–1698.

20. Beecher HK. Relationships of significance of wound to pain experienced. *JAMA* 1956;161(17):1609–1613.

21. Carroll LJ, Holm LW, Ferrari R, Ozegovic D, Cassidy JD. Recovery in whiplash-associated disorders: do you get what you expect? *J Rheumatol* 2009;36(5):1063–1070.

22. Beecher HK. The powerful placebo. *JAMA* 1955;159(17):1602–1606.

23. Levine JD, Gordon NC, Fields HL. The mechanism of placebo analgesia. *Lancet* 1978;2(8091):654–657.

24. Dum J, Herz A. Endorphinergic modulation of neural reward systems indicated by behavioral changes. *Pharmacol Biochem Behav* 1984;21:259–266.

25. Carvalho C, Caetano JM, Cunha L, Rebouta P, Kaptchuk TJ, Kirsch I. Open-label placebo treatment in chronic low back pain: a randomized controlled trial. *Pain* 2016;157:2766–2772.

26. Kam-Hansen S, Jakubowski M, Kelley JM, Kirsch I, Hoaglin DC, Kaptchuk TJ, Burstein R. Altered placebo and drug labeling changes the outcome of episode migraine attacks. *Sci Transl Med* 2014;6:218ra5.

27. Jensen KB, Kaptchuk TJ, Chen X, Kirsch I, Ingvar M, Gollub RL, Kong J. A neural mechanism for nonconscious activation of conditioned placebo and nocebo responses. *Cerebral Cortex* 2015;25:3903–3910.

28. Marras W, Davis K, Heaney C, Maronitis A, Allread W. The influence of psychosocial stress, gender, and personality on mechanical loading of the lumbar spine. *Spine* 2000;25(23):3045–3054.

29. Fuentes J, Armijo-Olivio S, Funabashi M, Miciak M, Dick B, Warren S, Rashiq S, Magee DJ, Gross DP. Enhanced therapeutic alliance modulates pain intensity and muscle pain sensitivity in patients with chronic low back pain: an experimental controlled study. *Phys Ther* 2014;94(4):477–489.

30. Kaptchuk TJ, Kelley JM, Conboy LA, Davis RB, Kerr CE, Jacobson EE, Kirsch I, Schyner RN, Nam BH, Nguyen LT, Park M, Rivers AL, McManus C, Kokkotou E, Drossman DA, Goldman P, Lembo AJ. Components of placebo effect: randomised controlled trial in patients with irritable bowel syndrome. *BMJ* 2008;336(7651):999–1003.

31. Dossett ML, Mu L, Davis RB, Bell IR, Lembo AJ, Kaptchuk TJ, Yeh GY. Patient-provider interactions affect symptoms in gastroesophageal reflux disease: a pilot randomized, double blind, placebo-controlled trial. *PLoS One* 2015;10(9):e0136855.

32. Derksen F, Bensing J, Lagro-Janssen A. Effectiveness of empathy in general practice: a systematic review. *Br J Gen Pract* 2013;63(606):e76–e84.

33. Hojat M, Louis DZ, Markham FW, Wender R, Rabinowitz C, Gonnella JS. Physicians' empathy and clinical outcomes for diabetic patients. *Acad Med* 2011;86(3):359–364.

34. Rakel DP, Hoeft TJ, Barrett BP, Chewning BA, Craig MB, Niu M. Practitioner empathy and the duration of the common cold. *Fam Med* 2009;41(7):494–501.

35. Ruben MA, Meterko M, Bokhour BG. Do patient perceptions of provider communication relate to experiences of physical pain? *Patient Educ Couns* 2018;101:209–213.

36. Bandura A. Self-efficacy. In Ramachaudran VS (Ed.), *Encyclopedia of Human Behavior* (Vol. 4). New York: Academic Press, 1994:71–81.

37. Hsiao-Wei Lo G, Balasubramanyam AS, Barbo A, Street RL, Suarez-Almazor ME. Link between positive clinician-conveyed expectations of treatment effect and pain reduction in knee osteoarthritis, mediated by patient self-efficacy. *Arthritis Care Res* 2016;68(7):952–957.

38. Rollnick S, Miller WR, Butler CC. *Motivational Interviewing in Health Care: Helping Patients Change Behavior.* New York: Guilford, 2008.

39. Miller WR. Motivational interviewing with problem drinkers. *Behav Psychother* 1983;11:147–172.

40. Tuccero D, Railey K, Briggs M, Hull SK. Behavioral health in prevention and chronic illness management: motivational interviewing. *Prim Care Clin Office Pract* 2016;43:191–202.

41. Chang YP, Compton P, Almeter P, Fox CH. The effect of motivational interviewing on prescription opioid adherence among older adults with chronic pain. *Perspect Psychiatr Care* 2015;51(3):211–219.

42. Vong SK, Cheing GL, Chan F, So EM, Chan CC. Motivational interviewing therapy in addition to physical therapy improves motivational factors and treatment outcomes in people with low back pain: a randomized controlled trial. *Arch Phys Med Rehabil* 2011;92:176–183.

43. Alperstein D, Sharpe L. The efficacy of motivational interviewing in adults with chronic pain: a meta-analysis and systematic review. *J Pain* 2016;17(4):393–403.

44. Cheing G, Vong S, Chan F, Ditchman N, Brooks J, Chan C. Testing a path-analytic mediation model of how motivational enhancement physiotherapy improves physical functioning in pain patients. *J Occup Rehabil* 2014;24:798–805.

45. Miller WR, Rollnick S. *Motivational Interviewing: Helping People Change.* 3rd ed. New York: Guilford Press, 2013.

46. Miller WR, Zweben A, DiClemente CC, Rychtarik RG. *Motivational Enhancement Therapy Manual: A Clinical Research Guide for Therapists Treating Individuals with Alcohol Abuse and Dependence.* Rockville, MD: National Institute on Alcohol Abuse and Alcoholism, 1992.

47. Miller WR, Rollnick S. Ten things that motivational interviewing is not. *Behav Cogn Psychother* 2009;37:129–140.

48. Beck A, Rush AJ, Shaw BF, Emery G. *Cognitive Therapy of Depression.* New York: Guilford Press, 1979.

49. Sullivan MJL, Thorn B, Haythornthwaite JA, Keefe F, Martin M, Bradley LA, Lefebvre JC. Theoretical perspectives on the relation between catastrophizing and pain. *Clin J Pain* 2001;17:52–64.

50. Thorn BE. *Cognitive Therapy for Chronic Pain: A Step-by-Step Guide.* 2nd ed. New York: Guilford, 2017.

51. Otis JD. *Managing Chronic Pain: A Cognitive-Behavioral Therapy Approach.* New York: Oxford University Press, 2007.

52. Melzack R, Wall PD. Pain mechanisms: a new theory. *Science* 1965;150:971–979.

53. Murphy JL, McKellar JD, Raffa SD, Clark ME, Kerns RD, Karlin BE. *Cognitive Behavioral Therapy for Chronic Pain Among Veterans: Therapist Manual.* Washington, DC: U.S. Department of Veterans Affairs.

54. Ehde DM, Dillworth TM, Turner JA. Cognitive behavioral therapy for individuals with chronic pain: efficacy, innovations, and directions for research. *Am Psychol* 2014;69(2):153–166.

55. Hayes SC, Barnes-Holmes D, Roche B (Eds.). *Relational Frame Theory: A Post-Skinnerian Account of Human Language and Cognition.* New York: Plenum Press, 2001.

56. Hayes SC. Acceptance and commitment therapy, relational frame theory, and the third wave of behavioral and cognitive therapies. *Behav Ther* 2004;35:639–665.

57. Hayes SC, Strosahl KD, Wilson KG. *Acceptance and Commitment Therapy: An Experiential Approach to Behavior Change.* New York: Guilford Press, 1999.

58. Harris R. *ACT Made Simple.* Oakland, CA: New Harbinger Publications, 2009.

59. Cherkin DC, Sherman KJ, Balderson BH, Cook AJ, Anderson ML, Hawkes RJ, Hansen KE, Turner JA. Effect of mindfulness-based stress reduction vs. cognitive behavioral therapy or usual care on back pain and functional limitations in adults with chronic low back pain: a randomized clinical trial. *JAMA* 2016;315(12):1240–1249.

60. Grant JA, Courtemanche J, Rainville P. A non-elaborative mental stance and decoupling of executive and pain-related cortices predicts low pain sensitivity in Zen meditators. *Pain* 2011;152(1):150–156.

61. Sharon H, Maron-Katz A, Ben Simon E, Flusser Y, Hendler T, Tarrasch R, Brill S. Mindfulness meditation modulates pain through endogenous opioids. *Am J Med* 2016;129(7):755–758.

Further Reading

Building Empathy

Coulehan JL, Platt FW, Egener B, Frankel R, Lin CT, Lown B, Salazar WH. "Let me see if I have this right ...": words that help build empathy. *Ann Intern Med* 2001;135(3):221–227.

Communication Strategies to Increase Patient Motivation

Miller WR, Rollnick S. *Motivational Interviewing: Helping People Change.* 3rd ed. New York: Guilford Press, 2013.
Rollnick S, Miller WR, Butler CC. *Motivational Interviewing in Health Care: Helping Patients Change Behavior.* New York: Guilford, 2008.

CBT and ACT for Chronic Pain

Harris R. *ACT Made Simple.* 2nd ed. Oakland, CA: New Harbinger Publications, 2009.
Otis JD. *Managing Chronic Pain: A Cognitive-Behavioral Therapy Approach.* New York: Oxford University Press, 2007.

3

The Patient Who Rates Pain as 14/10

Leanne R. Cianfrini

Case: "The Patient Who Rates Pain as 14/10"

What is your first reaction when a patient—a patient who drove to your office, sat in your waiting room, and exchanged pleasantries with the receptionist— rates their current pain a "10" on a scale of 0 to 10? What if the patient provides a "14/10" rating? Does your perspective change if the patient is relatively new to your practice? What if the patient is involved in litigation, is pursuing a social security or work-related long-term disability claim, or is covered under worker's compensation insurance? What if the patient is also wincing, moaning, and clutching at their back? What if the 10/10 rating comes after a series of opioid increases or your attempts at multiple interventional procedures?

Challenge: How to Interpret and Respond to Higher-Than-Expected Pain Ratings

When you are confronted with a higher-than-expected pain intensity rating, a common attribution may be:

This patient is exaggerating.

Further, we might suspect that the patient is exaggerating for a nefarious and intentional reason:

This patient is exaggerating for secondary gain of some sort, including increased medicine doses or for legal documentation.

A possible "knee-jerk response" might be to challenge the patient:

"You can't be a 14/10!"

Correcting the patient in such a blunt way conveys, "Your pain is not as bad as you say it is." "I don't trust your rating." "You are whining." "You're being dramatic." Any of those direct or indirect accusations from the provider could shut down communication immediately. Recall from Chapter 2 the clinical value of active listening and empathic responses. However, it is important to obtain accurate baseline and periodic ratings of pain intensity from the patient, especially given that higher pain severity ratings are significantly associated with both greater physician-reported visit difficulty[1] and higher opioid usage.[2]

Clinician Context: Clinical Decision-Making in the Face of Uncertainty Is Complicated and Prone to Unintentional Bias

As a clinician, you are familiar with reading results of laboratory tests. A patient who mistakenly says their hemoglobin A1C is 11.2 can be shown the bloodwork results to reset their understanding of the severity of their diabetes. Unfortunately, we simply do not have that same type of objective feedback for chronic pain. Diagnostic imaging scans (e.g., magnetic resonance imaging [MRI], computed tomography [CT] scans) or bloodwork (e.g., positive antinuclear antibody [ANA] or high C-reactive protein levels) do not "prove" the presence or severity of pain any more so than unremarkable tests "prove" that a patient is malingering.[3] Thus, health care providers working in the area of chronic pain must often make clinical decisions based on insufficient evidence, despite the expectation that they are practicing evidence-based medicine. In most acute pain conditions, medical evidence might play a more central role; however, judgments become less certain when pain persists for longer than expected and psychosocial factors become more salient correlates of pain and functional impairment.[4]

According to an excellent review article by Tait and colleagues,[5] "When symptom certainty is high, clinical judgments and resultant medical decisions are more straightforward, even when a clinical condition is complex.

When symptom certainty is low (i.e., the validity of a pain report is subject to question), however, clinical judgments are more ambiguous, and patients may be vulnerable to undertreatment" (p. 12). The literature suggests that clinicians, from medical students[6] to trained and experienced health professionals,[7] tend to underestimate pain in vignette assessments, especially in the face of a paucity of medical evidence. Propensity to discount higher pain ratings has been associated with clinician factors such as experience, as well as patient demographic variables such as older age, female gender, minority ethnic status, and dramatic demonstration of psychological distress.

In the absence of clear surgical pathology (which, to reiterate, does not "prove" pain), overt pain behaviors are sometimes used as a proxy for pain intensity. The term *pain behaviors* was coined by Fordyce in the 1970s[8] to encapsulate observable verbal (e.g., vocalizations of distress, moaning) and nonverbal (e.g., wincing, bracing, guarding) behaviors, but these are imperfect and subjective indicators as well. In clinical practice, we might see this phenomenon range from a patient who absentmindedly rubs his affected knee to a patient who dramatically clutches his back and cries out suddenly and loudly after slightly shifting in the seat while looking at you out of the corner of his eyes to see if you noticed.

Although attempts have been made to develop a reliable assessment of pain behaviors during functional examinations,[9] video-based assessment methods requiring extensive training are better suited for experimental, not clinical, conditions. There are conditions in which self-reports of pain intensity are positively correlated with observations of pain behaviors;[10] however, a recent study showed that individual differences in pain behaviors remained stable over time even when accounting for pain severity.[11] Earlier explanations for the persistence of pain behaviors in patients with chronic pain focused on possible operant reinforcement contingencies (e.g., empathic attention by clinicians or significant others to patient pain behaviors increases the likelihood of future pain behaviors).[8] More recent research has pointed to the partial influence of fear of movement,[11] pain catastrophizing (see later in the chapter for further discussion), and even long-term neuroplastic changes in central nervous system regions responsible for the motor programs involved in the overt expression of pain.[12] Just like higher-than-expected pain intensity ratings, whether intentional or unintentional, whether serving a function for attention, physical protection, or communication, whether influenced by psychosocial or neurophysiological factors, overt pain behaviors also do not "prove" pain. However, they can detract from effective patient–clinician interactions. In practice, we find that many patients are not aware of their own automated and stereotyped patterns of pain behaviors and can inhibit such behaviors when brought to their attention.

Patient Context: There Is a Range of Possible Explanations for Higher-Than-Expected Pain Ratings

Consider these possibilities:

- Our pain intensity rating scales are incomplete/insufficient to capture the patient experience.
- The patient does not fully understand how to use the pain intensity rating scale.
- The patient wants to convey, "I'm really suffering here and need you to believe me."
- The patient fears elimination of treatment (e.g., medication reduction, denial of further interventional procedures) if they report a "mild" or improved pain rating.
- The patient may be intentionally exaggerating for secondary gain.
- The patient may have a maladaptive belief style—catastrophizing—in which symptoms are magnified.

We will delve further into a few of these possibilities next.

Limitations to Clinical Assessment Utility and Patient Comprehension Are Inherent in Our Current Pain Intensity Rating Scales

Pain perception is a personal, covert process, and as mentioned earlier, there is no failsafe mechanical means of measuring an individual's pain experience. Many of our patients have lamented the lack of such an instrument of empathy: "I wish my doctor or my wife could feel what I feel for just 20 seconds so they'd know what I'm going through." Imagine that sense of isolation, knowing that traditional verbal communication is inadequate to share what you feel, why the pain seems like an insurmountable barrier to accomplishing your goals, why you're so desperate for compassionate and immediate care. In chronic pain especially, signs of overt autonomic arousal (e.g., increased blood pressure, perspiration) do not always correspond directly to pain intensity, so one must avoid "judging a book by its cover" during an office consultation. Quantitative sensory testing (QST) has been developed for use in experimental pain research settings (e.g., responses to thermal, mechanical, ischemic stimulation) and can illuminate some psychophysiological parameters in neuropathic pain states like an individual's pain threshold, tolerance, or degree of central sensitization, allodynia, or hyperalgesia.[13] However, QST is still dependent on patient self-report and is not feasible to implement in most busy clinical practices. That leaves us with quantified subjective measures to identify pain intensity at its worst, least, current, and average.

Let's touch briefly on the challenging nature of our current linear pain rating scales commonly used in office. Ratings scales for adults include numeric rating scales (NRSs), visual analog scales (VASs), and verbal rating scales.[14] The NRS is a unidimensional measure of pain intensity in adults, essentially a segmented numeric version of the VAS. Whereas the VAS has respondents create a perpendicular mark along a horizontal line representing their pain intensity, on the NRS patients are instead asked to select a number from 0 to 10 or 0 to 100. Similar to the VAS, the NRS is anchored by terms describing pain severity extremes (e.g., from "no pain" to "most intense pain imaginable"). Alternatives are available for children or adults who have communication difficulties, such as the Wong-Baker FACES Pain Scale,[15] among others. For examples of these scales, which are all available in the public domain, see Figure 3.1. These rating scales are generally reliable and valid, although there are some complicating factors to consider, such as the wording of the response anchors, cultural translatability, and ability to use the scale across paper versus electronic modes of data collection. The Initiative on Methods, Measurement, and Pain Assessment in Clinical Trials (IMMPACT) guidelines indicate that the NRS is the gold standard in measurement of pain intensity in adults without cognitive impairment,[16] and more recent broad literature reviews support that claim.[17]

To empathize with how difficult these scales might be for patients, consider some rhetorical questions: Is your 6/10 the same as your patient's

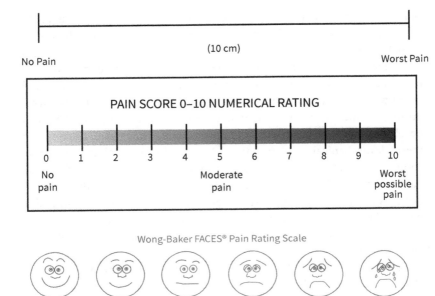

Figure 3.1 Three types of pain intensity rating scales[14,15]

6/10? Is their 10/10 anchor stable or dynamic across time and situation? If your patient experiences concurrent neck, lower back, *and* migraine pain, which location are they addressing when they give you the single numeric rating? Should multiple intensity ratings be generated for each pain site, or can pain intensity be accurately aggregated into a single number? Might their emotional distress or suffering affect the number they provide (e.g., are they sensitive and intuitive enough to rate pure intensity or is their rating affected by how unpleasant they find their pain)? Is the patient trying in an unsophisticated manner to convey something *more* by the number they provide?

Results from a recent study[18] highlight the limitations of using a single unidimensional pain rating in clinic paperwork. While controlling for pain intensity as measured by a NRS, higher scores on measures representing pain interference with function (perceived pain-related disability), pain catastrophizing, and pain-related beliefs such as a biomedical belief in a pain cure were all associated with a tendency for study participants to rate their pain as more severe on a verbal rating scale. Thus, pain severity ratings cannot necessarily be assumed to measure only pain intensity; they may also reflect the patient's perceptions about disability and other beliefs about pain. Experienced clinicians are well aware of the discrepancy between subjective pain ratings and objective measures of function: patients who give similar pain intensity ratings may exhibit very different degrees of psychological and physical impairment.

So, our unidimensional pain intensity scales alone are an imperfect attempt to quantify a subjective, multidimensional, and dynamic experience. We recommend broadening the measurement of a patient's pain experience by incorporating tools to assess perceived pain-related limitations in activities of daily living by using an appropriate disability index relevant to the patient's condition. As we know, a focus on pain intensity may be a principal outcome, but only in the context of the patient's overall quality of life and function. Of course, validity of pain-related disability measures can also be questionable because of the self-report nature (e.g., we have had patients rate a sitting tolerance of only 10 minutes but proceed to sit through an hour-long interview or class), and daily activity diaries for improved short-term recall are not always feasible. The Pain Disability Index[19] is a short, widely used questionnaire that produces ratings of general pain limitations on obligatory and discretionary activities across seven functional content areas (e.g., family/home responsibilities, recreation, social life). Disease-specific functional instruments better reflect the impact associated with single disease states. For example, we use the Oswestry Disability Index[20] quite a bit in our practice, but these items (e.g., impact on lifting, sitting) were designed to measure disability in patients with low back pain and would not translate well to assess the unique functional and parafunctional interference possible with head and facial pain, for example (e.g., impact on chewing, yawning, creating facial expressions of emotion). In those circumstances, indices like the Jaw Functional Limitations Scale[21] or the Migraine Disability Assessment Scale[22] would be more suitable.

As conceptualized eloquently by D. A. Williams,[23] "if you are listening to music, knowing only the volume setting tells you little about instrumentation, quality, key or tempo of the piece that is being played." In other words, we need to go *beyond the 0-to-10 scale* and consider additional aspects of the patient's experience, such as the unpleasantness or "suffering" component. We could use an additional VAS or NRS in our paperwork to capture the "pain unpleasantness" dimension. Alternately or in conjunction, the McGill Pain Questionnaire (MPQ)[24] can be used not only to evaluate the sensory component of pain, but also to capture qualities of the affective/emotional dimension of pain. The measure presents several groups of adjectives ranked in terms of severity, and can be administered as a paper-and-pencil test or by an evaluator reading each subclass of words. Studies have shown that the MPQ is able to discriminate among discrete clinical pain conditions, such as between migraine and tension-type headache.[25] Two validated short forms are now available.[26,27] Clinicians can use the information from the MPQ to guide interventions. For example, a patient who endorses several affective pain descriptors of high intensity (i.e., "terrifying," "unbearable," "vicious") may respond to treatment that targets pain anxiety, maladaptive pain beliefs, unrealistic expectations, or coping mechanisms. This plan may differ from a medical or behavioral treatment program designed for a patient who primarily endorses sensory descriptors such as "aching," "tender," and "cramping," in which techniques such as non-opioid medications, nutritional supplementation, or muscle relaxation may be more suitable. We will discuss the utility of adding other measures of pain-related mood and beliefs in other chapters.

We also recommend educating the patient about the NRS or VAS scale used in your office. Simply dividing an NRS into arbitrary discrete categories or equal parts is not a valid method. One recommendation is to correlate pain intensity to the level of pain-related interference with daily functioning. This statistical approach has been repeated for cancer patients,[28] patients with musculoskeletal pain,[29] and other patient samples. In general,[30] studies show that the cutoff between "mild" and "moderate" pain in terms of pain-related interference with functioning is usually placed between 3 and 4. The cutoff between "moderate" and "severe" pain is usually between 6 and 8, depending on study samples, pain definitions, measures of interference/functioning, and pain diagnosis. During the required pain class at our clinic, we teach patients these general cutoffs before they even have their first evaluation with the physician. We teach them how to tie numeric ratings to function and pain flares and what defines the anchors (e.g., "If you rate that you are a 10/10 at your appointment, you might not have a very active imagination for what might be worse," "We will not chase a 0/10 pain rating at the expense of your safety"). We ask, "What number on that scale would be tolerable to you most days?" The average NRS intensity our clinic patients seem willing to tolerate is a very reasonable 5.2/10. Anecdotally, they wish for more consistent or predictable baseline pain within a moderate range, and a structure to support them during pain intensity flares. Feedback from our patients trained on the NRS scale has been positive and many have noted that they plan to re-anchor and reframe their intensity ratings based on the education. Patients have expressed gratitude at the opportunity to enhance communication with their clinician.

Patients' Fear of Provider Reactions or Prescribing Behaviors Might Drive Their Ratings

In our class discussions of the pain rating scale, two common threads have emerged as reasons for selecting higher pain ratings other than pain intensity itself. Many of our incoming patients have been through multiple previous clinicians (e.g., primary care physicians, orthopedists, rheumatology specialists, neurologists) and often feel "passed off" and "disbelieved." Anecdotal commentary suggests that some patients might give high pain ratings in an unsophisticated attempt to communicate the high impact of their chronic pain to their new provider.

A second theme has been that some patients fear elimination of treatment (e.g., medication reduction, insurance denial of additional epidural blocks) if they report a pain reduction to a rating in the "mild" category. For example, with opioid indications for "daily moderate to severe pain," one interpretation is that patients who report mild pain will no longer qualify for medication management rather than the opposite logic—that is, the medication is part of the toolset helping their pain settle to that mild rating. We teach them that providing inflated pain ratings could lead to dangerous or expensive medical outcomes (e.g., unnecessary diagnostic testing, increased dosing, termination of helpful therapies). We coach our patients not to play three-dimensional chess—in other words, we urge them to be direct, honest, and thoughtful about the pain intensity ratings and any questionnaire responses they provide. We ask them not to attempt to anticipate what the clinician might think or do. We assign them the task of being a responsible and accurate "scientist-observer" of their own pain.

The Patient May Be Intentionally Exaggerating for Secondary Gain

In some cases, the patient's credibility may be questioned, especially in instances in which significant financial incentives or other "secondary gain" advantages are involved (e.g., worker's compensation, ongoing litigation, disability applications, release from responsibilities at home, attention from family members or the medical community). Although data are mixed as to whether compensation patients exaggerate pain-related symptoms, many clinicians view such patients with skepticism.[31] We certainly have had a few patients who were well aware of how the promise of financial or social reward influenced their pain ratings and were surprisingly open about it—for instance, "My lawyer told me to keep my pain ratings high so I could get a bigger settlement," "My husband ignores me, except when I'm crying out in pain."

Factitious disorder and malingering are rare in clinical practice[32] and as such may be missed in the pain medicine setting. These non-organic syndromes may present as pain and/or neurologic complaints, with intentional fabrication or feigning of physical symptoms, or exaggerated expression of physical conditions in order to adopt a sick role. However, confirming these diagnoses requires difficult exclusions, including the following:

Conversion disorder (functional neurologic disorder)—report of neurologic sensory or motor symptoms not attributable to any medical condition and causing distress or impairment

Somatic symptom disorder—one or more somatic symptoms accompanied by excessive thoughts, feelings, and/or behaviors related to the somatic symptoms. Somatic symptom disorder supplanted a host of diagnoses such as hypochondriasis, somatoform disorders, and pain disorder in the latest version of the *Diagnostic and Statistical Manual of Mental Disorders*.[33]

Inferences about malingering must also be based on external data as well as clinician judgments about the patient's motives.

If your suspicion is getting the best of you, rather than jumping to conclusions or making judgments about a patient's motives, attempt through assessment methods to screen for symptom validity and level of effort/

motivation to identify the multiple driving forces behind patient motivation for symptom report. For example, the Modified Somatic Perception Questionnaire (MSPQ) and Pain Disability Index (PDI) are used in pain populations to differentiate between malingered pain-related disability and non-malingering patients.[34]

The Patient May Have a Maladaptive Belief Style (Catastrophizing) in Which Symptoms Are Magnified

Another explanation for high pain ratings involves a special type of distorted negative thinking, elucidated within the cognitive-behavioral perspective. You have seen a patient who is engaging in *pain catastrophizing* if you've heard the phrases, "My pain is killing me," "I can't think about anything other than pain," "I can't cope with this," and/or "My pain is always a 10 out of 10 and will never get better." Defined both as a maladaptive appraisal or coping style and a stable dispositional trait, pain catastrophizing is most readily defined by its three components:[35]

Magnification (amplified symptom perception)
Rumination (inability to direct attention away from painful sensations)
Helplessness (feeling unable to cope with the pain given one's present resources).

Pain catastrophizing is a particularly influential construct that has been shown to be a potent predictor of pain-related disability,[36] quality of life,[37] suicidal ideation,[38] observable pain behavior and spousal responses,[39,40] as well as postsurgical pain ratings and narcotic usage (e.g., [41]), often exceeding the contribution of depression itself to these outcomes. Relevant to our discussion of high intensity ratings, pain catastrophizing predicts pain intensity independent of the level of physical impairment.[42] A recent study[43] showed a significant interaction effect for pain catastrophizing and pain intensity on opioid prescriptions. Pain catastrophizing has also been implicated as a predictor for poor response to minimally invasive procedures such as radiofrequency lesioning and injection treatments,[44] as well as a predictor of persistent pain at two years following total knee arthroscopy.[45] Pain catastrophizing has been identified as a risk factor for prescription opioid misuse in patients with chronic pain generally[46] and among those with a history of substance use disorder.[47]

With regard to mechanism of action, there is recent evidence that catastrophizing affects supraspinal endogenous pain-inhibitory and pain-facilitatory processes (e.g., [48]) and is associated with dysfunctional cortisol responses (e.g., [49]), and it may be linked to altered neuroimmunologic responses to pain. Neuroimaging studies conducted on healthy volunteers have shown that pain catastrophizing is associated with amplified activity in areas of the brain associated with the experience of pain, and this directly correlates with report of increased pain.[50]

The silver lining is that pain catastrophizing is a construct that is responsive to both longer-course (e.g., [51]) and brief, targeted psychological treatment,[52,53] within group settings, and even within one single session. Given its powerful relationship with treatment outcomes, pain catastrophizing has been characterized as "a primary, high-yield therapeutic target."[54]

During the course of CBT with a pain psychologist, patients would be taught to monitor their thoughts, identify any irrational beliefs or thought distortions, and restructure their thought pattern toward more adaptive and realistic appraisals of the situation. For example, to "de-catastrophize," patients would be guided to evaluate the realistic probability of their worst-case imagined scenario and identify resources to cope with it. A therapist might ask, "What's the worst thing that could happen with your pain?", "How sure are you that this will occur?", and "If so, then what? Could you cope with that?" With a teamwork approach and techniques such as modeling, role-playing exercises, and a careful questioning dialog, therapist will assist patients with challenging their negative thoughts and encourage them to create alternatives. It is important to note that CBT is not about "putting on rose-colored glasses" or adopting a "Pollyanna personality," which is just as distorted as one who habitually thinks through a negative filter. Rather, the goal is to adopt a realistic and neutral view of the pain and other situations.

So, in a busy medical practice, we recommend that you first simply listen for phrases indicative of rumination, magnification, or helplessness that might enlighten you about the influence of catastrophizing on the pain rating scales. We also recommend using a simple and brief questionnaire like the Pain Catastrophizing Scale[35] in your intake and follow-up paperwork to further assess for this construct.

Communication: Using Higher-Than-Expected Pain Ratings to Guide Clinical Conversations

As we mentioned in the beginning of the chapter, our first gut reaction might be to counter the patient's high numerical rating: "It can't be a 14!" The instinct to reorient patients to more helpful ways of rating their pain intensity is not wrong: if patients want their pain to be taken seriously, they need to take the pain scales seriously. A delicate and respectful touch with the pain scale education can go a long way. In addition, there are other ways to respond that might be more therapeutic. Your selection of conversational prompts and procedures from the following suggestions will depend on the amount of time you have with the patient, the patient's health literacy, the goal for the patient's care, and of course, your own personal style.

What Not to Say

- "Your pain can't be a 14/10!"
- "You're clearly exaggerating."
- "You're being a bit dramatic, aren't you?"
- "I think you're faking it to get disability insurance approved."
- "Oh, you poor thing. You must be in so much pain if you're moaning like that."

General Suggestions for Improving Conversations About Pain Ratings

- Pause. Don't react with your first gut response.
- Remember that the 0-to-10 scale might be vague for most patients.
- Make sure the NRS or VAS on your clinic paperwork is anchored with clear guidance.
- Ask how the patient interprets "10/10—worst pain imaginable."
- Consider education about mild/moderate/severe pain categories tied to daily function.
- Ask what number on the scale the patient would define as "tolerable."

- Either ignore overt pain behaviors (don't reinforce with positive attention, alarm, or pity) or gently point them out once to see if the patient is aware and can alter posture or calm facial expressions.
- Consider the history and psychosocial context of the patient. Is the patient involved in litigation or other opportunities for secondary gain? Is this patient sophisticated in verbal communication about pain otherwise?
- Consider giving the MPQ to obtain an improved picture of pain descriptors and severity of both sensory and emotional components of the pain experience.
- Consider including the Pain Catastrophizing Scale as part of your clinic paperwork; high scores might explain the patient's high rating.

Suggested Phrases to Use

- *"So, you're rating your pain as pretty intense."*
  - This is a simple active listening technique of reflection, which conveys empathy without judgment. It's an accurate and genuine reflection of the patient rating.
- *"Can I discuss a more helpful way to use the 0-to-10 scale with you that will help us communicate better?"*
  - Asking "permission" is a technique used in motivational interviewing. It implies teamwork and opens the conversation up to education about your pain rating scale.
- *"Are you aware that your right shoulder is raised higher than the left? We call that a guarding posture. Try to drop that for me."*
  - This question and request can actually be diagnostic. For patients who are unaware of their pain behavior, you can ask them to try periodic body scans throughout the day to raise awareness and practice calming their posture or facial expression. If they are unable to relax the posture or calm the rubbing or wincing behavior when prompted, there might be an element of fear (e.g., "If I don't guard the back, someone might bump it and cause more pain") or secondary gain (e.g., "My pain is invisible and if I don't show that I hurt, how will my family know to leave me alone about the chores?").

- *"I've noticed that your pain score is staying exactly the same no matter what we do—blocks, medicine increases, physical therapy. What do you think is going on there?"*
  - Being direct with an observation might introduce further discussion to reveal secondary gain issues, unrealistic expectations for relief ("If I'm not a 0/10, I just say nothing's working"), patient fear of treatment withdrawal if they provide lower ratings, and so forth. Often, a nonjudgmental question that simply addresses "the elephant in the room" can enhance trust in the interpersonal relationship.
- *"Your high pain score tells me that we should work on reducing your level of distress about your pain. Distress like that, which is so common with chronic pain, is actually a pain amplifier and can get in the way of relief."*
  - This response validates and "normalizes" the patient's distress—it's true that many patients are distressed by their pain.
  - It signals that their distress isn't *causing* the pain, per se, but rather can make their pain worse. *Note*: You might need to clarify that you're *not* implying, "The pain is all in your head."
- *"Your score on one of our questionnaires suggests that your pain is being impacted by a particular negative mindset."*
  - Here, you're using patient-friendlier language ("negative mindset" or perhaps "unhealthy thought habit") rather than psychological jargon ("pain catastrophizing"). This helps enhance the patient's receptiveness to the treatment plan, which will likely involve referral to a pain psychologist for further cognitive–behavioral interventions for catastrophizing.
  - One helpful follow-up remark is, *"What's really amazing is that if we're able to shift this negative mindset into a healthier perspective, research shows that your medical treatments can actually work more effectively and your function improves!"*
  - To introduce the idea of working with a local pain psychologist for CBT, you can suggest *"adding another member of your healthcare team"* who can address this mindset directly. Describing the psychologist as a *"behavioral medicine specialist"* who *"helps you retrain your brain pathways"* might be more palatable to some patients who seem nervous or reluctant about mental health treatment.

References

1. Henry SG, Bell RA, Fenton JJ, Kravitz RL. Communication about chronic pain and opioids in primary care: impact on patient and physician visit experience. *Pain* 2018;159(2):371–379.

2. Ciccone DS, Just N, Bandilla EB, Reimer E, Ilbeigi MS, Wu W. Psychological correlates of opioid use in patients with chronic nonmalignant pain: a preliminary test of the downhill spiral hypothesis. *J Pain Symptom Manage* 2000;20:180–192.

3. Jensen CJ, Brant-Zawaszki MN, Obuchowski N, Modic MT, Malkasian D, Ross JS. Magnetic resonance imaging of the lumbar spine in people without back pain. *N Engl J Med* 1994;331:69–73.

4. Gatchel RJ, Dersh J. Psychological disorders and chronic pain: are there cause-and-effect relationships? In Turk DC, Gatchel RJ (eds.), *Psychological Approaches to Pain Management: A Practitioner's Handbook.* 2nd ed. New York: Guilford Press, 2002:30–51.

5. Tait RC, Chibnall JT, Kalauokalani D. Provider judgments of patients in pain: seeking symptom certainty. *Pain Med* 2009;10(1):11–34.

6. Chibnall JT, Tait RC, Ross L. The effects of medical evidence and pain intensity on medical student judgments of chronic pain patients. *J Behav Med* 1997;20:257–271.

7. Tait RC, Chibnall JT. Physician judgment of patients with intractable low back pain. *Soc Sci Med* 1997;45:1199–1205.

8. Fordyce WE. *Behavioral Methods for Chronic Pain and Illness.* St. Louis: CV Mosby, 1976.

9. Koho P, Aho S, Watson P, Hurri H. Assessment of chronic pain behaviour: reliability of the method and its relationship with perceived disability, physical impairment, and function. *J Rehab Med* 2001;33:128–132.

10. Labus JS, Keefe FJ, Jensen MP. Self-reports of pain intensity and direct observations of pain behavior: when are they correlated? *Pain* 2003;102:109–124.

11. Martel MO, Thibault P, Sullivan MJL. The persistence of pain behaviors in patients with chronic back pain is independent of pain and psychological factors. *Pain* 2010;151:330–336.

12. Apkarian AV, Bushnell MC, Treede RD. Human brain mechanisms of pain perception and regulation in health and disease. *Eur J Pain* 2005;9:463–484.

13. Walk D, Sehgal N, Moeller-Bertram T, Edwards RR, Wasan A, Wallace M, Irving G, Argoff C, Backonja MM. Quantitative sensory testing and mapping: a review of nonautomated quantitative methods for examination of the patient with neuropathic pain. *Clin J Pain* 2009;25(7):632–640.

14. Jensen NP, Karoly P. Self-report scales and procedures for assessing pain in adults. In Turk DC, Melzack R (eds.), *Handbook of Pain Assessment*. New York: Guilford Press, 2011:19–44.

15. Wong D, Baker C. Pain in children: comparison of assessment scales. *Pediatr Nurs* 1988;14(1):9–17.

16. Dworkin RH, Turk DC, Farrar JT, Haythornthwaite JA, Jensen MP, Katz NP, Kerns RD, Stucki G, Allen RR, Bellamy N, Carr DB, Chandler J, Cowan P, Dionne R, Galer BS, Hertz S, Jadad AR, Kramer LD, Manning DC, Martin S, McCormick CG, McDermott MP, McGrath P, Quessy S, et al. IMMPACT core outcome measures for chronic pain clinical trials: IMMPACT recommendations. *Pain* 2005;113(1-2):9–19.

17. Safikhani S, Gries KS, Trudeau JJ, Reasner D, Rüdell K, Coons SJ, Buch EN, Hanlon J, Abraham L, Vernon M. Response scale selection in adult pain measures: results from a literature review. *J Patient Rep Outcomes* 2018; 2: 40.

18. Jensen MP, Tome-Pires C, de la Vega R, Galan S, Sole E, Miro J. What determines whether a pain is rated as mild, moderate, or severe? The important of pain beliefs and pain interference. *Clin J Pain* 2017;33(5):414–421.

19. Pollard CA. Preliminary validity study of the Pain Disability Index. *Perceptual and Motor Skills* 1984;59:974.

20. Fairbank JC, Couper J, Davies JB, O'Brien JP. The Oswestry Low Back Pain Questionnaire. *Physiotherapy* 1980;66(8):271–273.

21. Ohrbach R, Larsson P, List T. The Jaw Functional Limitation Scale: development, reliability, and validity of 8-item and 20-item versions. *J Orofac Pain* 2008;22-23:219–230.

22. Stewart WF, Lipton RB, Dowson AJ, Sawyer J. Development and testing of the Migraine Disability Assessment (MIDAS) questionnaire to assess headache-related disability. *Neurology* 2001;56(6, suppl. 1):S20–S28.

23. Williams DA. The importance of psychological assessment in chronic pain. *Curr Opin Urol* 2013;23(6):554–559.

24. Melzack R. The McGill Pain Questionnaire: major properties and scoring methods. *Pain* 1975;1:277–299.

25. Mongini F, Deregibus A, Raviola F, Mongini T. Confirmation of the distinction between chronic migraine and chronic tension-type headache by the McGill Pain Questionnaire. *Headache* 2003;43(8):867–877.

26. Dworkin RH, Turk DC, Revicki DA, Harding G, Coyne KS, Peirce-Sandner S, Bhagwat D, Everton D, Burke LB, Cowan P, Farrar JT, Hertz S, Max MB, Rappaport BA, Melzack R. Development and initial validation of an expanded and revised version of the Short-form McGill Pain Questionnaire (SF-MPQ-2). *Pain* 2009;144:35–42.

27. Katz JMR, Melzack R. The McGill Pain Questionnaire: development, psycho-metric properties, and usefulness of the long form, short form, and short form-2. In Turk DC, Melzack R (eds.), *Handbook of Pain Assessment*. New York: Guilford Press, 2011:45–66.

28. Paul SM, Zelman DC, Smith M, Miaskowski C. Categorizing the severity of cancer pain: further exploration of the establishment of cutpoints. *Pain* 2005;113:37–44.

29. Boonstra AM, Schiphorst Preuper HR, Balk GA, Stewart RE. Cut-off points for mild, moderate, and severe pain on the visual analogue scale for pain in patients with chronic musculoskeletal pain. *Pain* 2014;155(12):2545–2550.

30. Hirschfeld G, Zernikow B. Variability of "optimal" cut points for mild, mod-erate, and severe pain: neglected problems when comparing groups. Pain 2013;154:154–159.

31. Tait RC. Compensation claims for chronic pain: effects on evaluation and treat-ment. In Dworkin RH, Breitbart WS (eds.), *Psychosocial Aspects of Pain: A Handbook for Health Care Providers*. Seattle, WA: IASP Press, 2004:547–570.

32. Bass C, Halligan PW. Factitious disorders and malingering: challenges for clin-ical assessment and management. *Lancet* 2014;383(9926):1422–1432.

33. American Psychiatric Association. *Diagnostic and Statistical Manual of Mental Disorders*. 5th ed. Arlington, VA: American Psychiatric Association, 2013.

34. Bianchini KJ, Aguerrevere LE, Guise BJ, Ord JS, Etherton JL, Meyers JE, Soignier RD, Greve KW, Curtis KL, Bui J. Accuracy of the Modified Somatic Perception Questionnaire and Pain Disability Index in the detection of malingered pain-related disability in chronic pain. *Clin Neuropsychol* 2014;28(8)1376–1394.

35. Sullivan MJ, Bishop SR, Pivik J. The Pain Catastrophizing Scale: development and validation. *Psychol Assessment* 1995;7:524–532.

36. Severeijns R, Vlaeyen JW, van den Hout MA, Weber WE. Pain catastrophizing predicts pain intensity, disability, and psychological distress independent of the level of physical impairment. *Clin J Pain* 2001;17(2):165–172.

37. Lame IE, Peters ML, Vlaeyen JW, Kleef M, Patijn J. Quality of life in chronic pain is more associated with beliefs about pain, than with pain intensity. *Eur J Pain* 2005;9:15–24.

38. Edwards RR, Smith MT, Kudel I, Haythornthwaite J. Pain-related catastrophizing as a risk factor for suicidal ideation in chronic pain. *Pain* 2006;126:272–279.

39. Sullivan MJ, Adams H, Sullivan ME. Communicative dimensions of pain catastrophizing: social cueing effects on pain behavior and coping. *Pain* 2004;107(3):220–226.

40. Keefe FJ, Lefebvre JC, Egert JR, Affleck G, Sullivan MJ, Caldwell DS. The relationship of gender to pain, pain behavior, and disability in osteoarthritis patients: the role of catastrophizing. *Pain* 2000;87(3):325–334.

41. Roth ML, Tripp DA, Harrison MH, Sullivan M, Carson P. Demographic and psychosocial predictors of acute perioperative pain for total knee arthroplasty. *Pain Res Manag* 2007;12(3):184–194.

42. Severejins R, Vlaeyen JW, van den Hout MA, Weber WE. Pain catastrophizing predicts pain intensity, disability, and psychological distress independent of the level of physical impairment. *Clin J Pain* 2001;17(2):165–172.

43. Sharifzadeh Y, Kao MC, Sturgeon JA, Rico TJ, Mackey S, Darnall BD. Pain catastrophizing moderates relationships between pain intensity and opioid prescription: non-linear sex differences revealed using a learning health system. *Anesthesiology* 2017;127(1):136–146.

44. Van Wijk RM, Geurts, JW, Lousberg R, Wynne HJ, Hammink E, Knape JTA, Groen GJ. Psychological predictors of substantial pain reduction after minimally invasive radiofrequency and injection treatments for chronic low back pain. *Pain Med* 2008;9(2):212–221.

45. Forsythe ME, Dunbar MJ, Hennigar AW, Sullivan MJ, Gross M. Prospective relation between catastrophizing and residual pain following knee arthroplasty: two-year follow-up. *Pain Res Manag* 2008;13(4):335–341.

46. Martel MO, Wasan AD, Jamison RN, Edwards RR. Catastrophic thinking and increased risk for prescription opioid misuse in patients with chronic pain. *Drug Alcohol Depend* 2013;132:335–341.

47. Morasco BJ, Turk DC, Donovan DM, Dobscha SK. Risk for prescription opioid misuse among patients with a history of substance use disorder. *Drug Alcohol Depend* 2013;127:193–199.

48. Weissman-Fogel I, Sprecher E, Pud D. Effects of catastrophizing on pain perception and pain modulation. *Exp Brain Res* 2008;186(1):79–85.

49. Johansson AC, Gunnarsson LG, Linton SJ, Bergkvist L, Stridsberg M, Nilsson O, Cornefjord M. Pain, disability and coping reflected in the diurnal cortisol variability in patients scheduled for lumbar disc surgery. *Eur J Pain* 2008;12(5):633–664.

50. Seminowicz DA, Davis KD. Cortical responses to pain in healthy individuals depends on pain catastrophizing. *Pain* 2006;120(3):297–306.

51. Turner JA, Anderson ML, Balderson BH, Cook AJ, Sherman KJ, Cherkin DC. Mindfulness-based stress reduction and cognitive behavioral therapy for chronic low back pain: similar effects on mindfulness, catastrophizing, self-efficacy, and acceptance in a randomized controlled trial. *Pain* 2016;157(11):2434–2444.

52. Darnall BD, Sturgeon JA, Kao MC, Hah JM, Mackey SC. From catastrophizing to recovery: a pilot study of a single-session treatment for pain catastrophizing. *J Pain Res* 2014;7:219–226.
53. Thorn BE, Pence LB, Ward LC, Kilgo G, Clements KL, Cross TH, David AM, Tsui PW. A randomized clinical trial of targeted cognitive behavioral treatment to reduce catastrophizing in chronic headache sufferers. *J Pain* 2007;8(12):938–949.
54. Darnall BD, Colloca L. Optimizing placebo and minimizing nocebo to reduce pain, catastrophizing, and opioid use: a review of the science and an evidence-informed clinical toolkit. *Int Rev Neurobiol* 2018;139:129–157.

Further Reading

Clinical Judgments in Chronic Pain

Tait RC, Chibnall JT, Kalauokalani D. Provider judgments of patients in pain: seeking symptom certainty. *Pain Med* 2009;10(1):11–34.

Pain Behaviors

Martel MO, Thibault P, Sullivan MJL. The persistence of pain behaviors in patients with chronic back pain is independent of pain and psychological factors. *Pain* 2010;151:330–336.

Pain Assessment

Fillingim RB, Loeser JD, Baron R, Edwards RR. Assessment of chronic pain: domains methods, and mechanisms. *J Pain* 2016;17(9 Suppl):T10–T20.

Pain Catastrophizing

Quartana PJ, Campbell CM, Edwards RR. Pain catastrophizing: a critical review. *Expert Rev Neurother* 2009;9(5):745–758.

Malingering

Bass C, Halligan P. Factitious disorders and malingering in relation to functional neurological disorders. *Handb Clin Neurol* 2016;139:509–520.

4

The Patient Who Says, "I Can't Do What I Used to Do"

Leanne R. Cianfrini

Case: "I Would If I Could, But I Can't So I Won't' "

Do these statements sound familiar to you?

- "I miss attending church services. I just can't sit through that hour anymore."
- "I feel isolated because I can't golf with my friends anymore."
- "I'm so embarrassed. My house is a pigsty because I can't clean up to my standards anymore."
- "I don't know why you keep pushing exercise, Doc. It's hard enough getting out of bed and taking a shower. I used to be a jogger, but you should spend one day with my pain. There's no way I can exercise!"
- "Yes, I know I shouldn't rest in my recliner so much, but I can't stand for more than five minutes."
- "I want the old me back."

Challenge: How to Reconceptualize "I Can'ts" in a Manner That Fosters, Not Hinders, the Therapeutic Alliance

Take a moment to reread those statements. Reflect on what they have in common. Every clinician has felt the prickle of frustration in the face of a "Yes, but ..." or an "I can't." Whether we realize it or not, we have goals for patients that we'd like them to reach. We all would benefit from movement, eating a healthy diet, avoiding sedating medications, engaging in social activities, and so on. When we present an instructional suggestion to a patient, it springs out of our fund of evidence-based knowledge, with the intent to help. If that recommendation is met with resistance, it somehow feels like either a personal attack on our expertise or an indicator that "This patient just doesn't WANT to get better." The phrase "I can't" just *feels* resistant. It *feels* defeatist.

We may retreat and stop giving suggestions, chalking the patient up as a lost cause. Our tone might get clipped and blame may be conveyed inadvertently. Or we may lean toward being a superficial cheerleader—"Yes, you can! Just think positive!"—which can also minimize the patient's experience of pain. Imagine that the patient has thrown a large concrete barrier in our path toward a goal and we're left pushing against it—an exhausting mental process. (By the way, that's often what *they* feel when pushing against the barrier of intractable pain.) So, we present here a few different ways of managing the "I can'ts" and the "Yes, buts." This involves a gentler approach that can spare us irritation and enrich the therapeutic alliance rather than leaving us exhausted and stuck behind that barrier.

When we look deeper at the statements from the beginning of the chapter, the common threads involve a sense of loss:

A sense of comparing one's life now to how it was before and coming up short in the process

A sense of a dividing line between the eras of "BP" and "AP" (before pain and after pain), with a fallacy of "life BP was all roses" and "life AP is all gloom"

A sense of reluctance to engage in a new way of living out of fear of pain, perhaps, or fear of failure, or a number of other conscious or subconscious reasons.

Some of these perceived losses are grounded in reality (e.g., "I've had a multi-level lumbar fusion and I can no longer enjoy my favorite hobby of bungee jumping"). Other perceived losses are rooted more in unwillingness to endure potential pain caused by engaging in a previous daily routine. One concept that resonates with patients is that their "I can'ts" can be addressed within the framework of grief. Indeed, narrative accounts from individuals seeking help from pain clinics suggest that grief over material, socioeco-nomic, functional, and personal losses is a prominent issue.[1]

Clinician Context: Recognizing Grief as a Valid But Modifiable Barrier

Consider the reaction to the death of a loved one—we experience the loss of their physical presence, perhaps the loss of a source of emotional support, the loss of routine in caregiving or social interactions, the loss of the imagined future with that person. Now, transfer that grief experience to the multifa-ceted cascade of losses accrued by a person with chronic pain from injury or degenerative conditions.[1,2] Patients may miss their physical fitness, spon-taneity, the ability to plan ahead and be reliable, social interactions, engage-ment in stress-relieving physical hobbies, the routine involved with work, financial stability, their imagined future as a person without a chronic illness. Subthemes also include philosophical losses such as identity and hope.[3,4] Researchers have identified parallel processes of grieving independent of the type of loss, whether the loss is that of a close relative or subsequent to chronic pain.[5]

As clinicians working with grieving patients, we first must recognize that there is no single way to grieve.[6] Would you agree that it is reasonable to ex-perience a range of emotions, altered behaviors, and/or negative thoughts for some time period after a loss? While the death of a close loved one is obvious and is often recognized by attention and support from others, with chronic pain the loss might be partial and less obvious, might elicit less sup-port from others ("disenfranchised grief"),[7] and is not finite. Nonfinite loss involves grief that persists and changes as aspects of life continually fall short of expectations.[8] Individuals with chronic illness and disability face ongoing discordance between their goal aspirations and physical reality—they may continually feel like they are falling short of expectations.

In addition, there is an even more complex challenge at the heart of grieving pain-related losses: ambiguity.[9] An ambiguous loss of a loved one might involve the case of a missing or abducted family member or when we as a caregiver watch our loved one lose cognitive capacity during the pro-gression of Alzheimer's dementia. The other person exists in a state that is simultaneously "there" and "not there." With regard to chronic pain, the lack of clarity about prognosis (i.e., none of us can really predict whether pain will last with 100% certainty or if a certain surgery or medication will provide relief) and fluctuating abilities create this state of ambiguity. So, a potential future without pain is simultaneously "possible" and "not possible," making discussions about acceptance of the "not possible" all the more challenging. In clinical practice, we notice this seems especially true in patients with relapsing-remitting conditions.

Recognizing and addressing grief in our patients with chronic pain becomes especially salient due to the association between prolonged grief related to chronic illness and greater use of hospital-based services (e.g., more frequent emergency room visits and longer hospital stays).[10] By expressing compassion for the patient within this dynamic and complicated grieving framework, and remembering that it is more effective to learn about and respect the patient's functional goals rather than impose our own, we can set a new tone for motivation and chart a new therapeutic course to get both clinician and patient over or around those treatment barriers.

Patient Context: Working Through Grief and Challenging Unhelpful Thoughts

Grieving and Acceptance

We have moved beyond the sequential stage model of the widely cited Kübler-Ross framework of the five stages of grief.[11] We understand now that the stages are not experienced in a linear fashion; rather, individuals move in and out of the phases across minutes, hours, weeks, or months, with emotions shifting along the way. In the stage of denial, the individual with chronic pain is in a state of shock and unable to confront the diagnosis or the potential longevity and persistence/chronicity of the symptoms. Comments indicative of this stage might be, "This pain isn't going to last; we just haven't found the cure yet" or "My doctor is wrong: I don't have fibromyalgia." This denial may be detrimental for patients with chronic pain because they may take a passive approach to care and not seek appropriate treatments. Conversely, denial of chronicity can set up a scenario of putting "all the eggs into one basket" for increasingly invasive procedures or non–evidence-based treatments as potential cures.

Anger may set in once a person realizes that resisting the diagnosis will not change the diagnosis. Conversations may be characterized by a sense of injustice ("This isn't fair! I don't deserve this!," "Why me?") or projection onto health care providers ("You need to fix this!"). Anger is a common defense mechanism (see Chapter 9) and a normal emotion. However, it is necessary to channel anger in a healthy manner to motivate and reveal values rather than letting inappropriate anger expression to shut down lines of communication and cause further physiologic harm.

Bargaining phases usually do not last long, but they may involve a sense of desperation for life to be what it once was. We may recognize a sense of guilt (e.g., "If my CRPS heals, I promise I'll stop smoking") or spiritual pleading ("Please, God, don't let this ruin my life"). "What ifs" might take over the thought pattern. Emotions of depression and anxiety can appear deeply (see Chapters 7 and 8). Bereavement and major depression share many overlapping symptoms. Sadness and/or irritability, loss of pleasure, changes to daily habits and thought patterns, helplessness, and guilt can all be part of a grieving process.

The latest edition of the American Psychiatric Association's *Diagnostic and Statistical Manual of Mental Disorders* (DSM-5) abolished the bereavement exclusion applied to depressive symptoms lasting less than two months.[12] The exclusion was omitted, in part, to remove the implication that bereavement typically lasts only two months. In addition, it is notable that grief/bereavement responds to the same psychosocial and medication treatments as depression that is not related to bereavement. So, you should be prepared to refer to a local therapist patients who demonstrate prolonged or profound symptoms that resemble depression and are profoundly grieving their pain-related losses. This simple Swedish proverb captures the benefits of discussing one's emotional experience: "Shared joy is double joy; shared sorrow is half sorrow."

As patients confront their losses and shift toward acceptance, we may see them re-evaluate their roles, goals, abilities, and desires. The concept of acceptance is fraught with misunderstanding. When patients hear the term *acceptance*, they often confuse it with "being okay" with what happened, resigning themself to perpetual suffering, or "giving up." Patients worry that when it comes to pain, acceptance means "this is as good as it gets." Such negative connotations, if not debunked, can lead to even stronger resistance. We know that when we try to directly control our emotions, thoughts, and physical sensations, the problems can be exacerbated. Consider the paradoxical increase in thinking of the "pink elephant" when told to suppress the image of a pink elephant, or realizing how many times you touch your face when instructed not to do so. As therapist Carl Jung said, "What you resist not only persists, but will grow in size."

Instead, in the grief framework, acceptance is more about recognizing that the new reality is permanent, being willing to tolerate the present circumstances, and finding ways to adapt to the new reality. Specifically applied to chronic pain, several factors have been derived to explain acceptance, including (1) the acknowledgment that a cure for pain is unlikely and (2) a shift of focus away from pain to non-pain aspects of life.[13] Acceptance involves taking a *nonjudgmental* attitude toward pain sensations; rather than labeling pain as a negative or positive experience or attempting to improve self-efficacy and control, pain acceptance involves a willingness to have pain without taking action to eliminate it.[14] Behavioral medicine specialists often work within an acceptance and commitment therapy (ACT) framework to treat chronic pain. Recent meta-analyses have shown promising support for the use of ACT to impact a variety of chronic pain outcomes,[15,16] although more robust clinical trials are still needed.

Pursuit of Valued Activities

> "What one does is what counts. Not what one had the intention of doing."
>
> —Pablo Picasso

Chronic pain can impact movement in the direction toward a patient's values. *Values* are principles, morals, standards, or ideals that give our lives meaning, importance, and worth. They can be the guiding compass that drives our behavior and determines our goals. Some examples of values would include being physically fit, being a kind person, being trustworthy, being financially secure, being a good friend, being creative, or being a hard worker. To discover your core personal values, it can be helpful to ask what values you were honoring at the time of a peak, meaningful experience. What must you have in your life to experience fulfillment? What would you most like your friends to say about you at your funeral?

Patients often describe feeling "stuck" in their grief, in their disrupted routines, or in their suffering. "I can't do what I used to do" implies that a patient was engaging in a valued activity and now perceives pain as a barrier blocking movement toward that value. A behavioral medicine therapist working within the ACT orientation would discuss goals not in direct problem-solving terms ("Yes, you CAN do this, and here's how!") but rather in terms of helping patients to recognize core personal values, define life activities consistent with these values, work to reduce pain-related and other barriers toward pursuit of values, and engage in patterns of "committed action" linked to their chosen values.[17]

Committed action involves a goal-directed, psychologically flexible persistence. For individuals living with chronic pain, persistence with avoidance or overactivity behaviors can lead to greater disability and distress.[18,19] The standard therapeutic approach when avoidance or overexertion cycles are recognized is to teach activity pacing, or breaking up behavior patterns into active segments and rest breaks. However, pacing as an intervention is often poorly defined[20] and thus difficult to study.

As an alternative, within the ACT framework, Harris[21] clearly outlines four steps to committed action:

1. Choosing a domain of life that is a high priority for change
2. Choosing the values you wish to pursue in that domain
3. Developing specific goals that are guided by those values
4. Taking action mindfully.

See Table 4.1 for an example of how one might work through this process.

Behavior patterns are viewed in this model as more persistent when linked to values and goals, flexible to accommodate failure and discomfort, and amenable to stopping when inconsistent with reaching one's goals.[22] Of course, when defining goals in this process, it is helpful to keep in mind the mnemonic for SMART goals: specific, meaningful, adaptive, realistic, and time-framed.

One analogy for these steps comes from Russ Harris, a general practitioner and a world-renowned ACT trainer who makes a host of ACT materials available on his website (www.actmindfully.com.au). He suggests that a "value" is like a direction you want to move in (e.g., west). Committed action is like actually traveling west. Goals are like the bridges or mountains you

Table 4.1 Example of committed action exercise

	Example 1	Example 2
Define your **value**.	"To be a supportive friend"	"To take care of myself"
Identify a single **goal** consistent with that value.	Arrange a weekend trip with my two best friends so we can spend quality time together	Improve my ability to decrease pain's negative influence on my life
List 3 specific **behaviors** that will assist you in achieving the goal.	1. I'll start going out to lunch or to coffee with a friend once a week.	1. I'll check in with myself every morning to determine my options for the day and how my actions are impacting the things I value.
	2. I'll save $10 per week in order to fund the trip.	2. I'll take a moment each day to practice mindfulness, not judging my sensations.
	3. I'll check online to find a travel location that's affordable where we'd like to go.	3. I'll do something that's important to me each week when pain is present, even if it is a small, easy action.

aim to cross. In other words, rather than staying stuck with a thought of, "My pain makes me a bad friend. *I can't* go hang out on Tuesday for Taco Night anymore," one might say, "Being a good friend is so important to me. I'll set small goals that will build me up so I can get back to enjoying Taco Night despite the pain." Clinicians can support patients effectively in a time-efficient and patient-centered manner by helping them identify a few of their most cherished values and set appropriate values-oriented goals. Let them know you'll check in on these goals at the next visit to share in the excitement of their progress.

Negative Thought Barriers to Activity

There are a few unhelpful and habitual ways of thinking that tend to lead toward a sense of helplessness and frustration with pain-related activity interference. There may be issues with "overgeneralization" (e.g., "I failed at this task due to pain. I'm a failure at everything!"). There is also often a sense of comparing to an "old self" (e.g., "I used to be able to do everything I wanted to" or "Before pain, my life was perfect") or to others one considers "better off" (e.g., "My brother is able to do what he wants to do with no problems"). However, the most relevant negative thought habits that play into "I can'ts" fall into one of these three categories: all-or-nothing thinking, shoulds and musts, and confusing inability with reluctance.

All-or-Nothing Thinking

All-or-nothing thinking refers to thinking in extremes in a black-and-white or binary way. It might be difficult for patients to see the shades of gray or options along the continuum of compromise; they may believe that anything short of 100% essentially equals 0%. This thought pattern can disrupt attempts to change toward healthier behavior or pursue goals despite pain. In a non–pain-related example, imagine a person who would like to follow a healthy diet. One small derailment (e.g., sneaking a donut hole at the office) may lead to the belief that one has totally failed, so why even try for the rest of the day?

In terms of pain and pursuit of activity, a patient might think, "Since I can't play the full eighteen holes of golf without pain like I used to, I won't go the course at all." The patient just sees two bad options: a life with no hobbies or engaging in hobbies that produce an increase to intolerable pain. As a clinician, you may also hear all-or-nothing thoughts creep into perspectives on medications—for instance, "I have to be on strong opioids or face intolerable pain and suffering." Patients may feel stuck within these no-win situations.

Shoulds and Musts

"Shoulds and musts" go by many names depending on the cognitive therapist you speak with: "rigid standards," "imperative thinking," "mustabatory thinking." We joke with some patients who can tolerate mild humor that "It sounds like you're 'should-ing' all over the place!" Whatever you call it, these are rigid, unbending rules that people set for themselves or others. A person who doesn't live up to these high, unrealistic expectations may feel guilty, and if someone else doesn't live up to the standard, the person might feel angry and resentful. These statements might take the form of the following:

"I shouldn't ask for help" (… and I can't do things on my own!)
"I should be able to do the laundry like I used to" (… and I can't do the laundry!)

"She ought to know how I feel and stop asking me to do things" (… because I can't do what she asks!)

Confusing "Inability" with "Reluctance" and "Having to" with "Choosing to"

One corollary to "should" statements is confusing "inability" with "reluctance." For most patients living with chronic pain who have functional limbs and reasonable resources, it is concern about pain itself that is the limiting factor. Patients who jump to "I can't" are likely underestimating their resources and not truly confronting the more honest statement of, "I could, but I'm reluctant to because of the potential for more pain." For example, a patient might tell you, "I *can't tolerate* a car ride of three hours." But, for the majority of patients, a three-hour (non–off-road) car ride might be tolerated with paced rest stops, use of pillows or heating pads, shifting positions, distraction during the trip, and planning a restful activity upon arrival. So, the "I can't" is actually shorthand for "I'm *reluctant to/nervous about/hesitant to* take a car ride because my pain *might* become intolerable."

The second related concept involves confusing "choosing to" and "having to": the person doesn't readily realize that something is a choice rather than a necessity—for example, "I *have to* give up fishing with my friends on Sundays because of pain" rather than "I *choose to* avoid fishing because I don't want to ask my friends to limit their hours or use a closer fishing spot."

Communication: Addressing Grief, Challenging Negative Thought Barriers, and Motivating Patients Toward Valued Goals

What Not to Say

- "Yes, you *can* do that. Knock it off!"
- "Stop whining."
- "I have back pain and I exercise four times a week, so there's no reason you can't."

General Suggestions for Improving Communication

- Listen for phrases that suggest grief, resistance, or thought distortions. Go back to the beginning of the chapter for examples of "I can'ts," "I shoulds," and "The old me . . ." You'll hear them.
- Use these phrases not as triggers for your own frustration as a clinician, but as a cue to open up a potentially important line of discussion with the patient.
- It might be particularly helpful to monitor for an increase in symptoms around the anniversary of a patient's injury, diagnosis, or major surgeries, or during holidays. It seems like grief tends to remember the milestones.
- If you notice profound or complicated grieving, consider making a referral to a local therapist.
- Check in first with your own emotions when you're encountering resistance before you react. "Rolling with resistance" is one of the key principles of motivational interviewing (MI), as mentioned in Chapter 2. Instead of fighting the resistance, follow it. Avoid a direct head-on argument, show that you've heard what the patient said, and encourage patients to come up with possible solutions or alternative behaviors themselves rather than forcing suggestions on them.

Suggested Phrases to Use

- **To open up the dialogue**: *"So you feel like you've lost your ability to socialize with your friends because of chronic pain. What do you see as some of your other losses?"*
  - Be prepared to hear common tangible losses (e.g., financial stability, energy, ability to engage in hobbies) but also losses to identity (e.g., self-esteem, confidence, ability to be a dependable person) and future plans.
- **To offer the grief framework**: *"It sounds like you're grieving these changes since pain came into your life."*

- Don't shy away from contextualizing the patient's comment under the umbrella of grieving—this can help to normalize what they're experiencing and provide a framework for emotional healing.
- **To use an empathic statement:** *"I'm so sorry you're going through that."*
  - When in doubt, a simple statement of empathy can build the therapeutic alliance.
- **To inquire about the patient's support system:** *"Do you have people in your life you can talk to about how you feel?"*
  - You can ask if they have friends, family, support of a religious community, or if they're involved in support groups already.
  - Depending on the severity of the symptoms, you can recommend online pain support communities like the American Chronic Pain Association (www.theACPA.org) or refer the patient to a local therapist.
- **To normalize pain-related grief:** *"Pain-related grieving is a process many people experience. You may have heard about the stages of grief, an emotional process with movement toward acceptance. We know this process can take a short time in some and a long time in others. There's not really a right or wrong way to do it. But I'd like you to consider ways to find your path now, not looking too much in the past to what you used to do, and not looking too much in the future, since we can't predict that. Do you think you can shift attention to what you can do now, in this moment, with the abilities and skills and even the limitations you may have?"*
- **To clarify pain acceptance:** *"You heard me use the term* pain acceptance. *I understand that can sometimes have negative meanings for patients* [you can ask what acceptance means to them]. *I want you to know that I'm not saying 'give up' or 'you'll never feel better.'"*
  - *"Pain acceptance means being willing to experience the sensations you have moment to moment. You don't have to like the sensations and you can't pretend they're not there. But we can acknowledge that the sensations exist without labeling them as good, bad, painful, horrible, etc."*
  - *"Another good part of acceptance is that it lets us really define what our values are and begin to live our lives consistent with those values, despite how we feel physically."*
- **To plant the seed toward values-based action:** *"Can you identify an area of your life that you'd like to work on?"* (Examples might be work,

family, parenting, spiritual, community, personal growth, leisure, education, romantic relationship, etc.)

- *"Okay, what is an **underlying value** of yours in that domain? For example, you mentioned that you can't clean your house like you used to because of pain and you liked to do that for your family. Do you consider keeping a tidy home a valuable part of your identity?"*
- **Develop discrepancy.** This is another key principle of MI. Once you've reflected back to them that keeping a tidy home is a value, you could gently point out that their resting and retreating behaviors are not consistent with such a cherished goal. You might show that you realize their concern about a pain increase if they *overdo* the cleaning, and ask them how avoiding the activity entirely fits in with their aim of providing a calm and uncluttered environment for the family.
- *"We know that when we act in a way consistent with our values, we are more motivated and feel better overall. What are some **specific goals** you can set so that you can fulfil your value of keeping a neat home for your family?"*
- *Tip*: Have a reminder poster in your office about **SMART goals**:

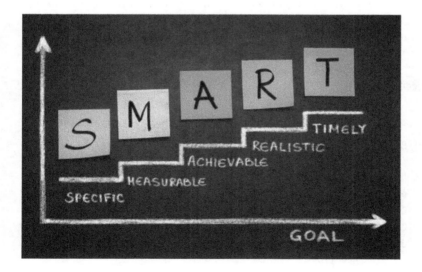

- **To challenge negative thought barriers to activity:**
  - *"So, you feel your pain prevents you completely from enjoying your gardening hobby. Sounds like your brain is setting up an either/or*

or all-or-nothing kind of situation: you either have to do your hobby exactly as you used to or you won't do it at all. Are there any 'shades of gray' between those black and white extremes? Are there any compromises you can propose so you can still do some gardening, either in a different way (modification) or paced throughout the week or season (moderation)?"

- *"You feel like you should be able to clean your house, walk your dog, work a full day, cook for the kids, and be a perfect wife and mother. Well, it sounds like you're should-ing all over the place! Those are some really high expectations you have for yourself, especially since it's also helpful to make time to listen to your body. What if you choose a few of those things you would really like to do and focus on those first? Be kind to yourself and challenge your thoughts whenever you catch yourself saying those shoulds."*

- *"I hear you saying 'I can't drive four hours to the beach because of my pain.' Sometimes, we say 'I can't' when what we really mean is 'I'm reluctant to make this drive because I might experience more pain afterward.' What would need to happen and what can you do to make that four-hour drive? Finish this sentence: I could do the drive if . . ."*

References

1. Furnes B, Dysvik E. Dealing with grief related to loss by death and chronic pain: an integrated theoretical framework. Part 1. *Patient Prefer Adherence* 2010;4:135–140.

2. Furnes B, Dysvik E. Dealing with grief related to loss by death and chronic pain: an integrated theoretical framework. Part 2. *Patient Prefer Adherence* 2010;4:163–170.

3. Gatchel RJ, Adams L, Polatin PB, Kishino ND. Secondary loss and pain-associated disability: theoretical overview and treatment implications. *J Occup Rehabil* 2002;12(2):99–110.

4. Walker J, Sofaer B, Holloway I. The experience of chronic back pain: accounts of loss in those seeking help from pain clinics. *Eur J Pain* 2006;10(3):199–207.

5. Parkes CM. *Bereavement: Studies of Grief in Adult Life.* London: Penguin, 1986.

6. Hart J. Moving through loss: addressing grief in our patients. *Altern Complement Ther* 2012;18(3):145–147.

7. Doka KJ. Disenfranchised grief in historical and cultural perspective In Stroebe MS, Hansson RO, Schut H, Stroebe W (eds.), *Handbook of Bereavement Research and Practice: Advances in Theory and Intervention.* Washington, DC: American Psychological Society, 2008:223–240.

8. Bruce EJ, Schultz CL. *Nonfinite Loss and Grief: A Psychoeducational Approach.* Baltimore: Paul H. Brookes Publishing, 2001.

9. Boss P, Couden B. Ambiguous loss from chronic physical illness: clinical interventions with individuals, couples, and families. *Psychotherapy in Practice* 2002;58(11):1351–1360.

10. Holland JM, Graves S, Klingspon KL, Rozalski V. Prolonged grief symptoms related to loss of physical functioning: examining unique associates with medical service utilization. *Disabil Rehabil* 2016;38(3):205–210.

11. Kübler-Ross E, Kessler D. *On Grief and Grieving: Finding the Meaning of Grief Through the Five Stages of Loss.* New York: Scribner, 2014.

12. American Psychiatric Association. *Diagnostic and Statistical Manual of Mental Disorders: Diagnostic and Statistical Manual of Mental Disorders.* 5th ed. Arlington, VA: American Psychiatric Association, 2013.

13. Risdon A, Eccleston C, Crombez G, McCracken L. How can we learn to live with pain? A Q-methodological analysis of the diverse understandings of acceptance of chronic pain. *Social Sci Med* 2003;56(2):375–386.

14. McCracken LM, Vowles KE. Acceptance of chronic pain. *Curr Pain Headache Rep* 2006;10(2):90–94.

15. Soler AF, Montesinos F, Gutierrez-Martinez O, Scott, W, McCracken LM, Luciano JV. Current status of acceptance and commitment therapy for chronic pain: a narrative review. *J Pain Res* 2018;11:2145–2159.

16. Hughes LS, Clark J, Colclough JA, Dale E, McMillan D. Acceptance and commitment therapy (ACT) for chronic pain: a systematic review and meta-analyses. *Clin J Pain* 2017;33(6):552–568.

17. Dahl JC, Wilson KG, Luciano C, Hayes SC. *Acceptance and Commitment Therapy for Chronic Pain.* Reno, NV: Context Press, 2005.

18. Kindermans HPJ, Roelofs J, Goossens MEJB, Uijnen IPJ, Verbunt JA, Vlaeyen JWS. Activity patterns in chronic pain: underlying dimensions and associations with disability and depressed mood. *J Pain* 2011;12:1049–1058.

19. McCracken LM, Samuel VM. The role of avoidance, pacing, and other activity patterns in chronic pain. *Pain* 2007;130:119–125.

20. Gill JR, Brown CA. A structured review of the evidence for pacing as a chronic pain intervention. *Pain* 2009;3:214–216.

21. Harris R. *ACT Made Simple*. Oakland, CA: New Harbinger Publications, Inc., 2009.

22. McCracken LM. Committed action: an application of the psychological flexibility model to activity patterns in chronic pain. *J Pain* 2013;14(8):828–835.

Further Reading

Acceptance and Commitment Therapy

- Harris R. *ACT Made Simple*. Oakland, CA: New Harbinger Publications, Inc., 2009.
- www.actmindfully.com.au

Online Support Group Recommendation

American Chronic Pain Association (ACPA): www.theacpa.org. This nonprofit organization offers an opportunity for patients with chronic pain to connect with a support group in their area or start their own. Educational modules on pain acceptance are readily available online.

5

The Patient Who Begs You to Fix Their Pain

Leanne R. Cianfrini

Case: The Patient Who Begs You to Fix Their Pain

What were your motives for entering a helping profession? Did you have a personal or family health experience that shaped your career goals? Regardless of the catalyst for your years of training and expenses, you are now in a position of authority and trust. What are your gut reactions when you hear a patient desperately plead, "Doc, you have to fix this!"? Do you have confidence "fixing" the disease of chronic pain? Do you feel a twinge of, "Oh no! This isn't all on me, buddy. It's a two-way street." How comfortable are you promoting patient self-management while remaining in the driver's seat for some of the critical health care decisions? This is a continuation of the discussion from Chapter 4—how to work with individuals who feel helpless to influence their own health, and in doing so shifts the bulk of the responsibility for their health care onto the clinician.

Challenge: How to Set Realistic Expectations and Shift to a Team Approach

The way we as clinicians speak with patients about their health care greatly influences their motivation for change toward healthier behaviors. Being able to skillfully mix listening, informing, and guiding communication skills is crucial to promoting behavior change. One of the first steps is to understand the patient's expectations for their pain outcomes and their role in long-term management.

Consider the following quotes about expectations:

"Expectation is the root of all heartache."—William Shakespeare
    "Expectations   are   premeditated   resentments."—Alcoholics
Anonymous
    "The secret of happiness is low expectations."—Barry Schwartz

Those sound pretty dire, don't they? They imply that we should simply go through life without expectations for the future or adopt a pessimistic "expect the worst, hope for the best" attitude. The problem is, that's not how humans act. Expectations may be expressed by patients as:

1. **Ideals:** values, hopes and desires, or preferred outcomes related to the patient's views of the potential health care service. For example, "I hope that this epidural block fixes my neck pain completely."
2. **Normative expectations:** what should happen, derived from what the patient is told, is led to believe, or thinks they are entitled to receive from health services. For example, "I think the epidural block will give me about 60% relief for a few months based on what my doctor told me."
3. **Predicted expectations:** belief about what is likely or probable to result based on personal experiences, reported experiences of others, and other sources of knowledge such as the media. For example, "I don't think this epidural block will work; blocks didn't help at all for my mother and cousin."[1,2]

In the health care literature, we know that patients' expectations are viewed as a major determinant for satisfaction with outcomes. For example, discrepancy between expectations and actual outcomes portends lower satisfaction for lumbar surgical outcomes[3] and results of total knee arthroplasty.[4] Expectations have been shown to be strong predictors of outcomes of interdisciplinary pain management programs,[5] acupuncture for chronic pain,[6] and opioid analgesic benefit (e.g., [7]). Interestingly, positive expectancy effects are associated with activity in the endogenous pain modulatory system.[7–9]

The importance of expectations was underscored in a recent functional magnetic resonance imaging (fMRI) study examining self-reinforcing pain expectations, or a "self-fulfilling prophecy."[10] Essentially, the more pain a participant expected based on manipulated cues during an experimental heat task, the stronger the brain responded in pain processing areas such as the anterior cingulate cortex, insula, and thalamus. The stronger the brain response, the more pain the patient expected on a subsequent trial. Furthermore, researchers observed a confirmation bias in learning. That is, patients did not learn on subsequent trials from evidence if it did not confirm what they already expected (i.e., they continued to predict high pain even if the previous stimulus was less intense than initially anticipated). This phenomenon has major implications for clinical treatment. A patient with a negative expectation (i.e., "This medicine won't work," "My pain won't respond to physical therapy") is fighting an uphill battle: not only will this negative expectation enhance perceived pain but it might also prevent them from noticing that they are actually getting better.

Identifying and meeting patients' expectations should result in more satisfaction with care,[11] which in turn might increase compliance, which in turn can foster even better pain management outcomes.[12,13] Setting expectations early in the therapeutic relationship is a unique opportunity for us as clinicians to be a catalyst for such a positive cycle. For an excellent discussion of the neurobiological underpinnings of positive expectancies for pain relief (you know this also as the "placebo effect") and expectations for persistent or worsening pain (aka the "nocebo effect"), the reader is referred to the 2018 article by Darnall and Colloca,[14] who also provide strategies on how to optimize these effects in clinical care.

Patients do not always voice their expectations unprompted, especially their desires for referrals or physical therapy.[15] Patient expectations can differ widely from those of their clinicians,[16] and failure to clarify expectations remains a blind spot in clinical care. In an international survey, although approximately 89% of clinicians believed it was important to ask patients about expectations, only 16% reported actually asking.[17] In a qualitative study, researchers found that patients living with chronic pain mostly desire to understand and have an explanation for their pain (i.e., pain "legitimized" through acknowledgment of a biological etiology) and to regain a sense of normality in their routines and activities.[18] Some patients desire a cure, while some are more accepting and desire reasonable long-term management.

Clearly, it is more challenging when patients are fixated on a cure and place that demand in your lap. In any of these situations, early clinical goals are to align patient expectations with what can realistically be achieved and to shift the balance of control from the pain (or from you) to the person living with the pain.

Clinician Context: Resist the Urge to Make Unrealistic Promises or To Persuade the Patient Toward a Particular Course of Action

Within the practice of motivational interviewing (MI), there are four guiding principles or "RULEs": Resist, Understand, Listen, and Empower. The first principle is to resist the "righting reflex." Although the directive to heal and prevent harm is right there in the Hippocratic Oath, following our first reflexive inclination to correct the patient's course through persuasion ("No, don't do it that way; do it this way!") can actually have a paradoxical effect. You've learned this the hard way if you've ever raised a teenager. In the social psychology realm, this resistance to the social influence of others is defined as "reactance"[19]—the motivation to regain a freedom after it has been lost or threatened. It's quite difficult to resist this urge to go for the dunk shot with paternalistic advice giving, especially if a patient is putting that ball right in your hands.

Reactance theory contrasts with the concept of learned helplessness, which is a state of passively enduring a threat or withdrawing from it ([20], also see Chapter 8). Reactant individuals, in contrast, have a strong urge to do something, but mostly want to change the threat to their freedom. Let's use as an example a recommendation for a patient undergoing spinal fusion to quit smoking. A patient who feels helpless might not quit smoking because they feel powerless to make the change, believe that they have low strength or low willpower, and are sure they will not be successful. A reactant individual may feel capable of quitting, but the desire to change the threat to their freedom becomes more potent (i.e., your imperative to quit smoking challenges their freedom of choice to smoke). One of the authors (LRC) vividly recalls a patient bursting into tears at the suggestion to reduce caffeine intake (from four liters of Diet Coke daily) to help with sleep onset. When asked about her emotional reaction, the patient said, "Pain has already taken so much away from me. I refuse to lose another thing!" She reacted strongly to the insinuated threat to her freedom to drink Diet Coke, even though she recognized it as an unhealthy behavior.

These reactance behaviors become particularly aroused in the face of forceful persuasive messages. Terms such as "should," "must," and "need" are perceived as more threatening and elicit more reactance than noncontrolling language such as "consider," "can," "could," and "may."[21,22] Furthermore, messages framed as loss (e.g., "You'll lose mobility if you don't exercise") are seen as more threatening and are associated with more anger than messages framed as gains (e.g. "If you find a way to exercise, you can gain mobility and a better quality of life").[23]

In a "shared medical decision-making" model, the collaborative process between clinician and patient integrates the patient's preferences and expectations as well as joint decision-making. For example, a patient may indicate a strong preference to avoid surgery or to avoid a side effect of nausea. In this framework, the patient and clinician would work together to identify and select a treatment plan that best matches the patient's preferences. Of note, some patients may not want this sort of relationship with their clinician. Patients who are younger, female, and well educated are more likely to engage their clinicians in shared medical decision-making.[24] We also need to be aware of potential biases in whom we approach with this model: there is evidence that clinicians are less likely to be collaborative with patients from lower socioeconomic groups or from ethnic minority groups.[25,26] For an excellent review on shared medical decision-making in the management of chronic pain, the reader is directed to the 2007 article by Frantsve and Kerns.[27]

So, rather than simply using the power of persuasion, a better place to start is finding out where the patient is coming from in terms of their expectations. Then, empathize with and empower the patient to take steps toward change by affirming their strengths and eliciting *their* initiative to participate in their self-care. Treatment decisions can be made in a collaborative manner to enhance outcomes and patient satisfaction if the patient desires to share in the process.

Patient Context: I Feel Helpless or Lack Confidence in the Face of My Pain and Need Guidance from My Trusted Physician

Health-Related Locus of Control

One of the factors driving a patient's request that you lead the way in their treatment may be related to their general sense of who's ultimately responsible for their health or illness. Health-related locus of control (HLOC) is a term that refers to an individual's perception of the factors that control their health.[28] The "locus" suggests the location where control is thought to reside—either internally or externally. Locus of control is an individual difference construct originally derived from Rotter's social learning theory.[29] The primary measure of HLOC, the Multidimensional Health Locus of Control questionnaire,[30] has three subscales delineating belief in (a) external locus of control due to chance or luck, (b) external locus of control due to "powerful others," such as health care providers, or (c) internal locus of control. Internal HLOC refers to one's tendency to believe that health outcomes are principally due to one's own behavior, willpower, or sustained efforts. Questionnaire responses have been used to predict or explain health behaviors across a variety of health conditions. This table summarizes some general HLOC research:

High Internal HLOC	High Powerful Others HLOC	High Chance HLOC
More likely to seek health-related information[28]	More trust in health professionals[37]	More passive and maladaptive coping approaches[39,40]
Higher survival rates after lung transplant[31]	Associated with hostility and passive coping[38]	Higher likelihood of smoking, less attention to healthy nutrition[35]
More likely to return to work after coronary artery bypass surgery[32]		Rate abilities to control pain as poor[40]

High Internal HLOC	High Powerful Others HLOC	High Chance HLOC
More likely to engage in preventive health behaviors (e.g., dental care, smoking cessation, weight loss, flu shots, seatbelt use, exercise)[33,34]		Higher scores on depression scales and general psychological distress[40,41]
Willingness to use health smartphone apps and on-line health trackers [35]		
Predictor of reduced pain in a multidisciplinary inpatient treatment program for chronic pain[36]		

Consistent with the theory of planned behaviors,[42] an individual's beliefs about their ability to control their health are associated with willingness to engage in behaviors that could improve their health. HLOC may be an influential factor in the success of health interventions as it reflects intrinsic (regulated by personal interest and satisfaction) or extrinsic (regulated by compliance, rewards, and punishments) motivation toward participation in treatment.[43] We understand that it can become overwhelming to try to juggle all of these personality, cognitive, social, and psychological factors that determine a patient's actions. It will be impossible to measure or ask about each patient's personal locus of control, level of helplessness, potential for reactance, expectations, and source of motivation. It is, however, helpful to simply realize that there are many complex and dynamic reasons for a patient to ask you to fix their pain before you react.

Pain Self-Efficacy

The most recently researched construct related to HLOC is self-efficacy. Self-efficacy was originally defined as "belief in one's capabilities to organize and execute the course of action required to produce given attainments."[44] This concept was explained in more depth in Chapter 2. In research addressing the role of self-efficacy in the context of chronic pain, self-efficacy relates to an individual's confidence in their ability to control or manage pain symptoms, fatigue, and functional changes.[45] The primary measure of self-efficacy in the context of pain is the widely used Pain Self-Efficacy Questionnaire (PSEQ).[46] There is even a fairly robust two-item short form of the PSEQ[47] that measures a patient's confidence in their ability to do some form of housework or pain/unpaid work and ability to live a normal lifestyle despite the pain. Such a brief tool could be more useful in clinical settings, with scores of 5 or less suggesting the patient might need help to improve their confidence to perform daily activities in the presence of pain. Pain self-efficacy is a robust correlate of key chronic pain outcomes (e.g., pain severity, mood distress, functional impairment) across multiple studies [see [48] for a meta-analytic review]. As such, low pain self-efficacy can be an important risk factor and high efficacy a protective factor.

The good news is that pain self-efficacy is amenable to improvement through interventions, even those not specifically targeted at self-efficacy. For example, cognitive-behavioral therapy and mindfulness-based stress reduction interventions for chronic pain can improve self-efficacy scores.[49] Self-efficacy can also respond to education and exercise interventions for patients with knee and hip osteoarthritis[50] and for patients with chronic musculoskeletal pain and depression.[51] As mentioned in Chapter 2, a clinician can help a patient develop self-efficacy in several ways:

1. Encourage the patient to set small, achievable, and measurable goals to help improve their sense of personal mastery.
2. Describe your experiences with other patients who have experienced success to utilize positive social modeling forces.
3. Use positive persuasive language when describing treatment options.
4. Help the patient work around their mood state to reinterpret negative expectations or bias.

Communication: Teaching "Life Hacks" and Promoting "Change Talk"

Pain Self-Management

In addition to shared decision-making, we can also accomplish the goals of person-centered care and an enhanced sense of self-efficacy through self-management support. Pain self-management is conceptualized as a set of tasks and processes that are used by a patient to maintain wellness in the presence of ongoing pain.[52] Some clinicians and patients view this set of skills as "life hacks" for individuals living with chronic pain. The Institute of Medicine defines self-management of chronic pain as involving (a) adherence to medical treatment, (b) managing personal, family, and social roles and responsibilities through cognitive and behavioral strategies, and (c) managing emotional consequences of conditions associated with chronic pain.[53]

Self-management is a well-accepted, highly effective component of care for diabetes mellitus, a condition similar to chronic pain in terms of its complexity and need for long-term management rather than simply finding a "cure."[54] Common components across various randomized controlled trials of chronic pain self-management programs include psychological training, lifestyle modification, pain education, physical activity, and mind–body therapy.[55] Meta-analytic reviews show modest long-term effects of self-management training programs on pain and disability in patients with chronic musculoskeletal conditions[55] and low back pain.[56] Such programs have also been developed as a cost-effective way to boost self-efficacy in low-income and low-literacy primary care patients with chronic pain.[57]

The concept of a pain "toolbox" or "toolkit" can be a simple and helpful framework to get started in a busy practice when you're faced with a patient who feels "stuck." Consider running educational videos in your waiting room or holding periodic seminars to educate patients about pain pathways and the role of the brain in pain. Our patients have responded very well to education in layperson's terminology about the gate control theory, descending modulation and the "drug cabinet in the brain," and neuroplasticity to demonstrate that they have some control over how they perceive and react to pain. This is also a great opportunity to utilize and recommend community resources and information technology resources. For example, there are some excellent, brief YouTube videos about these topics that you can link to on your website[58,59] to set the tone for your patients.

A pain self-management toolkit can also include suggestions for distractions and techniques for tolerating mood reactions and pain flares. Handouts for grounding techniques, visualizations, mindfulness exercises, and breath awareness can be useful tools. There are a variety of high-quality smartphone apps to use for guided relaxation, which are explored in more depth in Chapter 8. When given a chance, you can guide the patient away from use of strong pain language and worst-case scenario predictions. Of course, tangible modalities can also be included in the toolkit. Patients can be encouraged to create a physical location (a drawer or a box) to store their heating pads, acupressure devices, topical analgesics, physiotherapy exercise diagrams, social support phone numbers, essential oils for aromatherapy, and so on. Education about healthy eating and sleep hygiene also falls under the umbrella of pain self-management through lifestyle modification. Finally, patients welcome guidance on planning for pain flares and how to manage setbacks. Providing these practical approaches to pain care that are relatively easy to implement in the clinic setting helps both clinician and patient shift away from reliance on prescription opioid therapy. Beth Darnall's *The Opioid-Free Pain Relief Kit* is a well-written, useful book promoting patient self-management.[60]

Motivation

> *Motivation is a fire from within.*
> *If someone else tries to light that fire under you,*
> *chances are it will burn very briefly.*
> —Stephen R. Covey (1932–2012)

As described in Chapter 2, MI is a communication strategy used to help the patient shift toward adopting positive health behaviors by tapping into their own intrinsic motivation for change. MI has been associated with increased self-efficacy, with modest effects on compliance.[61,62] As a set of communication tools—not a fancy technique—MI can be used among your other strategies at each visit to improve patient outcomes. Use open-ended questions (i.e., questions that can't simply be answered by a yes or no) to elicit narrative responses from the patient. Reinforce any "change talk" you recognize to help the person move from simply contemplating change to preparing for and acting on that change.

This communication style sprung out of the work done by Prochaska and DiClemente on the transtheoretical model and stages of change,[63] which identifies a range of motivational phases. They are highlighted in the following list, along with some examples of patient comments defining each phase:

1. **Precontemplation**—"People are telling me I have to learn to live with the pain, but I don't want to." "It's not fair that I have pain. Why should I have to change my lifestyle?"
2. **Contemplation**—"I've heard that relaxation techniques can help with pain, but I'm so tense there's no way they will work for me." "Losing weight and learning better body mechanics might help, but that's way too much to take on right now."
3. **Preparation**—"I'm ready to learn new ways of coping with my pain." "I'd like to discuss what options are available for me to try, Doc."
4. **Action**—"I'm learning some good ways to keep my pain from interfering with my hobbies." "I can get busy livin' now despite my pain."
5. **Maintenance**—"I've been enjoying some new hobbies I found that I can do despite my pain."
6. **Relapse**—"I was plugging along with my new routine, but I had a pain flare that sent me back to square one. Why even try?"

So, your patients will come in at some point along these stages. What you say influences where they end up. A person with chronic pain who is expecting a cure may very well be in the precontemplation stage, not even ready to think about adopting a self-management approach to chronic pain. So, keep in mind that when patients say, "You need to fix my pain problem" or "No matter what people say about learning to live with the pain, I shouldn't have to ... there's a fix out there. My doctors just have to find it," they are stuck in an earlier stage of change. Different change strategies may be most effective at different points along the continuum (Figure 5.1). Practical strategies are offered next.

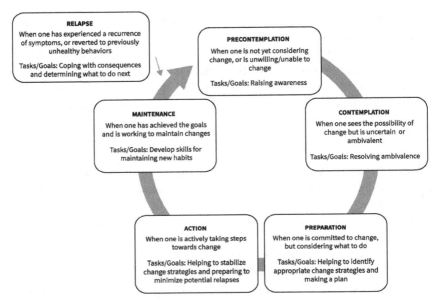

Figure 5.1 Stages of change and associated tasks

General Suggestions

- Calm the urge to persuade, especially with forceful "should/must" language. Resist the "expert trap."
- Start by setting a shared agenda for the appointment: "*Mrs. Smith, I'd like to review the results of your latest blood work with you, but what would you like to discuss today?*" This promotes the setting of shared decision-making.
- Prepare the patient for managing persistent pain by using "management" rather than "cure" language.
- Ask open-ended questions to elicit "change talk."
- Frame suggestions as a "gain" (e.g., "*When you reduce smoking, you gain benefits of improved oxygen to the tissues*") rather than a loss (e.g., "*If you don't give up smoking, you won't heal well from surgery*").
- Ask permission to share information: "*May I share with you some information about how exercise can help with musculoskeletal pain?*" Chances

are a patient won't say "no" to this, and this little step goes a long way toward promoting a sense of teamwork and respect. If they do refuse to hear your information, this is a cue to where they may be along the stages of change.

- Create opportunities for your patients to learn chronic pain self-management strategies through your website, waiting room videos, and handouts.

Suggested Phrases

- As mentioned, for behavior change to occur, the patient must feel that the change is important, must have motivation, and must feel capable (self-efficacy) to make the change. Try some "ruler questions" to gauge these conditions—they only take a minute and give a world of information.
  - *"How important would you say it is for you to be able to get back to work [or manage pain, or play soccer with your kid] on a scale of 0 to 10, with a 10 being extremely important?"* Why are you at a _____ and not zero? What would it take for you to go from _____ to a higher number?"
  - *"How confident are you that you can make this change, on a scale of 0 to 10, with a 10 being extremely confident?"* You can also ask "ruler questions" about desire for an outcome and commitment to an action.
- **Emphasize personal choice.** It's okay to state the obvious, but this shifts the ultimate decision-making to the patient about how compliant they will be with recommendations. Emphasizing patient choice helps to reduce reactance to perceived threats to their freedom of choice. For example, *"It seems like you don't have a great or easy choice here. We have to wait on a knee replacement until you get a little older, so we're left with medications, injections, exercise, or to just do nothing. When it comes down to it, what you do is really up to you."*
- Try to help the patient **look forward:** *"What will happen if things continue as they are?" "How would you like your life to be this time next year?" "If this treatment were 100% successful, what in your life would be different?"*

- Use **evocative questions** to encourage the patient to speak and use change talk: *"Remind me again the reasons you wanted to get the headaches under control."*
- Guide them through a **decisional balance** exercise: *"What are the pros and cons of keeping things the same with your opioid use and what are the pros and cons of trying a new path of tapering the opioids?"*
- Use **check-in questions** to see how the patient is responding to new information you've given them: *"What's your reaction to that?"*
- **Capitalize on** "change talk" when you hear it: *"So, you've toyed with the idea of a gym membership for exercise. What do you think you will do now?"* or *"Now that you have all the information on the table about why you want to start exercising to improve your core spine strength, what are you going to do now?"*
- Try an **ask—tell—ask** method:
  - **Ask** the patient what they already know or want to know about their pain: *"Mrs. Smith, what's your understanding of how degenerative disc disease leads to pain?"*
  - **Tell** the patient what they need to know. Hint: asking permission to share information with the patient helps to foster a sense of their control. *"May I share with you what we understand about degenerative disc disease from the medical perspective? DDD is not a fatal process and doesn't mean your spine is crumbling. Discs that are drying up can lessen the spine's ability to absorb shocks and cause less space for nerves to freely transmit information."*
  - **Ask** whether the patient understands the condition" *"Can you repeat that back to me in your own words?"* This part "closes the loop," helps the patient stay involved in the conversation, and gives you an opportunity to correct any misunderstandings.

References

1. Thompson AG, Sunol R. Expectations as determinants of patient satisfaction: concepts, theory and evidence. *Int J Qual Health Care* 1995;7:127–141.
2. Kravitz RL. Patients' expectations for medical care: an expanded formulation based on review of the literature. *Med Care Res Rev* 1996;53:3–27.

3. Witiw CD, Mansouri A, Mathieu F, Nassiri F, Badhiwala JH, Fessler RG. Exploring the expectation-actuality discrepancy: a systematic review of the impact of preoperative expectations on satisfaction and patient reported outcomes in spinal surgery. *Neurosurg Rev* 2018;41(1):19–30.

4. Noble PC, Conditt MA, Cook KF, Mathis KB. The John Insall Award: Patient expectations affect satisfaction with total knee arthroplasty. *Clin Orthop Relat Res* 2006;452:35–43.

5. Cormier S, Lavigne G, Choiniere M, Rainville P. Expectations predict chronic pain treatment outcomes. *Pain* 2016;157(2):329–338.

6. Linde K, Witt CM, Streng A, Weidenhammer W, Wagenpfeil S, Brinkhaus B, Willich SN, Melchart D. The impact of patient expectations on outcomes in four randomized controlled trials of acupuncture in patients with chronic pain. *Pain* 2007;128:264–271.

7. Bingel U, Wanigasekera V, Wiech K, Mhuircheartaigh R, Lee MC, Ploner M, Tracey I. The effect of treatment expectation on drug efficacy: imaging the analgesic benefit of the opioid remifentanil. *Sci Transl Med* 2011;3(70):70ra14.

8. Eippert F, Bingel U, Schoell ED, Yacubian J, Klinger R, Lorenz J, Büchel C. Activation of the opioidergic descending pain control system underlies placebo analgesia. *Neuron* 2009;63(4):533–543.

9. Pecina M, Zubieta JK. Expectancy modulation of opioid neurotransmission. *Int Rev Neurobiol* 2018;138:17–37.

10. Jepma M, Koban L, van Doorn J, Jones M, Wager TD. Behavioural and neural evidence for self-reinforcing expectancy effects on pain. *Nature Human Behaviour* 2018;2:838–855.

11. Barbosa CD, Balp MM, Kulich K, Germain N, Rofail D. A literature review to explore the link between treatment satisfaction and adherence, compliance, and persistence. *Patient Prefer Adherence* 2012;6:39–48.

12. Albrecht G, Hoogstraten J. Satisfaction as a determinant of compliance. *Community Dent Oral Epidemiol* 1998;26:139–146.

13. Haanstra TM, Kamper SJ, Williams CM, Spriensma AS, Lin CW, Maher CG, de Vet HCW, Ostelo RWJG. Does adherence to treatment mediate the relationship between patients' treatment outcome expectancies and the outcomes of pain intensity and recovery from acute low back pain? *Pain* 2015;156:1530–1536.

14. Darnall BD, Colloca L. Optimizing placebo and minimizing nocebo to reduce pain, catastrophizing, and opioid use: a review of the science and an evidence-informed clinical toolkit. *Int Rev Neurobiol* 2018;139:129–157.

15. Bell RA, Kravitz RL, Thom D, Krupat E, Azari R. Unsaid but not forgotten: patients' unvoiced desires in office visits. *Arch Intern Med* 2001;161(16):1977–1984.

16. Heisler M, Vijan S, Anderson RM, Ubel PA, Bernstein SJ, Hofer TP. When do patients and their physicians agree on diabetes treatment goals and strategies, and what difference does it make? *J Gen Intern Med* 2003;18(11):893–902.

17. Rozenblum R, Lisby M, Hockey PM, Levitizion-Korach O, Salzberg CA, Lipsitz S, Bates DW. Uncovering the blind spot of patient satisfaction: an international survey. *BMJ Qual Saf* 2011;20(11):959–965.

18. Bhana N, Thompson L, Alchin J, Thompson B. Patient expectations for chronic pain management. *J Prim Health Care* 2015;7(2):130–136.

19. Brehm JW. *A Theory of Psychological Reactance.* New York: Academic Press, 1966.

20. Seligman MEP. *Helplessness: On Depression, Development and Death.* San Francisco: Freeman, 1975.

21. Miller CH, Lane LT, Deatrick LM, Young AM, Potts KA. Psychological reactance and promotional health messages: the effects of controlling language, lexical concreteness, and the restoration of freedom. *Human Communication Research* 2007;33:219–240.

22. Quick BL, Stephenson MT. Examining the role of trait reactance and sensation seeking on perceived threat, state reactance, and reactance restoration. *Human Communication Research* 2008;34:448–476.

23. Cho H, Sands L. Gain- and loss-frame sun safety messages and psychological reactance of adolescents. *Communication Research Reports* 2011;28:308–317.

24. Ende J, Kazis L, Ash A, Moskowitz MA. Measuring patients' desire for autonomy. *J Gen Intern Med* 1989;4:23–30.

25. Willems S, De Maesschalck S, Deveugele M, Derese A, De Maeseneer J. Socioeconomic status of the patient and doctor–patient communication: does it make a difference? *Patient Edu Couns* 2005;56:139–146.

26. Ferguson WJ, Candib LM. Culture, language, and the doctor–patient relationship. *Fam Med* 2000;34:353–361.

27. Frantsve LME, Kerns RD. Patient-provider interactions in the management of chronic pain: current findings within the context of shared medical decision making. *Pain Med* 2007;8(1):25–35.

28. Wallston KA, Maides S, Wallston BS. Health-related information seeking as a function of health-related locus of control and health value. *J Res Pers* 1976;10:215–222.

29. Rotter JB. Generalized expectancies for internal versus external control of reinforcement. *Psychol Monogr* 1966;80:1.

30. Wallston KA, Wallston BS, DeVellis R. Development of the Multidimensional Health Locus of Control (MHLC) Scales. *Health Educ Monogr* 1978;6(2):160–170.

31. Burker EJ, Evon DM, Galanko J, Egan T. Health locus of control predicts survival after lung transplant. *J Health Psychol* 2005;10(5):695–704.

32. Bergvik S, Sorlie T, Wynn R. Coronary patients who returned to work had stronger internal locus of control beliefs than those who did not return to work. *Br J Health Psychol* 2012;17(3): 596–608.

33. Wallston BS, Wallston KA. Locus of control and health: a review of the literature. *Health Educ Monogr* 1978;6:107–117.

34. Helmer SM, Kramer A, Mikolajczyk RT. Health-related locus of control and health behaviour among university students in North Rhine Westphalia, Germany. *BMC Research Notes* 2012;5:703.

35. Bennett BL, Goldstein CM, Gathright EC, Hughes JW, Latner JD. Internal health locus of control predicts willingness to track health behaviors online and with smartphone applications. *Psychol Health Med* 2017;22(10):1224–1229.

36. Zuercher-Huerlimann E, Steward JA, Egloff N, von Kanel R, Studer M, Grosse Holtforth M. Internal health locus of control as a predictor of pain reduction in multidisciplinary inpatient treatment for chronic pain: a retrospective study. *J Pain Res* 2019;12:2095–2099.

37. Brincks AM, Feaster DJ, Burns MJ, Mitrani VB. The influence of health locus of control on the patient-provider relationship. *Psychol Health Med* 2010;15(6):720–728.

38. Brosschot JF, Gebhardt WA, Godaert GLR. Internal, powerful others, and chance locus of control: relationships with personality, coping, stress, and health. *Person Individ Diff* 1994;16(6):839–852.

39. Sørlie T, Sexton HC. Predictors of the process of coping in surgical patients. *Personality and Individual Differences* 2001;30(6):947–960.

40. Crisson JE, Keefe FJ. The relationship of locus of control to pain coping strategies and psychological distress in chronic pain patients. *Pain* 1988;35(2):147–154.

41. Wong HJ, Anitscu M. The role of health locus of control in evaluating depression and other comorbidities in patients with chronic pain conditions, a cross-sectional study. *Pain Pract* 2017;17(1):52–61.

42. Azjen I. The theory of planned behavior. *Organ Behav Hum Decis Process* 1991;50(2):179–211.

43. Ryan RM, Deci EL. Self-determination theory and the facilitation of intrinsic motivation, social development, and well-being. *Am Psychol* 2000;55:68–78.

44. Bandura A. Self-efficacy. In Ramachaudran VS (Ed.), *Encyclopedia of Human Behavior* (Vol. 4). New York: Academic Press, 1994:71–81.

45. Lorig K, Chastain RL, Ung E, Shoor S, Holman HR. Development and validation of a scale to measure perceived self-efficacy in people with arthritis. *Arthritis Rheum* 1989;32(1):37–44.

46. Nicholas MK. The pain self-efficacy questionnaire: taking pain into account. *Eur J Pain* 2007;11(2):153–163.

47. Nicholas MK. A 2-item short form of the pain self-efficacy questionnaire: development and psychometric evaluation of the PSEQ-2. *J Pain* 2015;16(2):153–163.

48. Jackson T, Wang Y, Wang Y, Fan H. Self-efficacy and chronic pain outcomes: a meta-analytic review. *J Pain* 2014;15(8):800–814.

49. Turner JA, Anderson ML, Balderson BH, Cook AJ, Sherman KJ, Cherkin DC. Mindfulness-based stress reduction and cognitive behavioural therapy for chronic low back pain: similar effects on mindfulness, catastrophizing, self-efficacy and acceptance in a randomized controlled trial. *Pain* 2016;157(11):2434–2444.

50. Jonsson T, Hansson EE, Thorstensson CA, Eek F, Bergman P, Dahlberg LE. The effect of education and supervised exercise on physical activity, pain, quality of life, and self-efficacy—an intervention study with a reference group. *BMC Musculoskeletal Disord* 2018;19(1):19.

51. Damush TM, Kroenke K, Bair MJ, Wu J, Tu W, Krebs EE, Poleshuck E. Pain self-management training increases self-efficacy, self-management behaviours and pain and depression outcomes. *Eur J Pain* 2016;20(7):1070–1078.

52. Lorig KR, Holman H. Self-management education: history, definition, outcomes, and mechanisms. *Ann Behav Med* 2003;26(1):1–7.

53. IOM (US) Committee on Advancing Pain Research Care, and Education. *Relieving Pain in America: A Blueprint for Transforming Prevention, Care, Education, and Research.* Washington, DC: National Academy of Sciences, 2011.

54. Beck J, Greenwood DA, Blanton L, Bollinger ST, Butcher MK, Condon JE, Cypress M, Faulkner P, Fischl AH, Francis T, Kolb LE, Lavin-Tompkin JM, MacLeod J, Maryniuk M, Mensing M, Orzeck EA, Pope DD, Pulizzi JL, Reed AA, Rhinehart AS, Siminerio L, Wang J. 2017 national standards for diabetes self-management education and support. *Diabetes Spectr* 2017;30(4):301–314.

55. Du S, Changrong Y, Xian X, Jing C, Yaoqin Q, Huijuan Q. Self-management programs for chronic musculoskeletal pain conditions: a systematic review and meta-analysis. *Patient Educ Couns* 2011;85(3):299–310.

56. Du S, Hu L, Dong J, Chen X, Jin S, Zhang H, Yin H. Self-management program for chronic low back pain: a systematic review and meta-analysis. *Patient Educ Couns* 2017;100(1):37–49.

57. Turner BJ, Liang Y, Simmonds MJ, Rodriguez N, Bobadilla R, Yin Z. Randomized trial of chronic pain self-management program in the community or clinic for low-income primary care patients. *J Gen Intern Med* 2018;33(5):668–677.

58. Davis K. *How Does Your Brain Respond to Pain?* https://www.youtube.com/watch?v=I7wfDenj6CQ

59. Butler D. *The Drug Cabinet in the Brain.* https://www.youtube.com/watch?v=Gd2NaGZa7M4

60. Darnall B. *The Opioid-Free Pain Relief Kit.* Boulder, CO: Bull Publishing Company, 2016.

61. Chang YP, Compton P, Almeter P, Fox CH. The effect of motivational interviewing on prescription opioid adherence among older adults with chronic pain. *Perspect Psychiatr Care* 2015;51(3):211–219.

62. Vong SK, Cheing GL, Chan F, So EM, Chan CC. Motivational interviewing therapy in addition to physical therapy improves motivational factors and treatment outcomes in people with low back pain: a randomized controlled trial. *Arch Phys Med Rehabil* 2011;92:176–183.

63. DiClemente CC, Prochaska JO. Toward a comprehensive, transtheoretical model of change: stages of change and addictive behaviors. In Miller WR, Heather N (Eds.), *Applied Clinical Psychology: Treating Addictive Behaviors.* New York: Plenum Press, 1998:3–24.

Further Reading

Doidge N. *The Brain That Changes Itself: Stories of Personal Triumph from the Frontiers of Brain Science.* New York: Viking, 2007.

Douaihy A, Kelly TM, Gold MA (Eds.). *Motivational Interviewing: A Guide for Medical Trainees.* New York: Oxford University Press, 2015.

Pain Toolkit: www.paintoolkit.org

Rollnick S, Miller WR, Butler CC. *Motivational Interviewing in Health Care: Helping Patients Change Behavior.* New York: Guilford, 2008.

For resources and webinars on motivational interviewing training for clinicians: https://www.integration.samhsa.gov/clinical-practice/motivational-interviewing

6

Discussions About Opioid Use

Leanne R. Cianfrini

Case: The Patient with Aberrant Drug Behaviors or the Patient Who Asks for Opioid Dose Increases in the Absence of Function

Review each of the following patient scenarios and assess whether you view it as a "red flag," a "yellow flag," or acceptable behavior in the context of your practice. Consider the patient who:

- Declines to get a recommended magnetic resonance imaging (MRI) scan to document new spinal pathology
- Delays participation in the recommended physical therapy, citing cost, transportation issues, or "It didn't fix the pain before"
- Says, "I've had pain for 20 years and I know that Roxicodone is the *only* pain medicine that works for me"
- Asks for one early refill because they are going on vacation and will be away from their pharmacy on the anticipated fill date
- Asks repeatedly for early refills for various reasons
- Indicates their function is worse on opioids
- Repeatedly takes more than the prescribed dose
- Fails to show up for a requested urine drug screen or pill count
- Fills an opioid prescription from three different physicians in the past month, per Prescription Drug Monitoring Program (PDMP) database information
- Informs you they spilled their remaining #30 tablets down the sink by accident
- Tells you, "This hydrocodone is not working. I can't do anything because of pain. I need more medicine."

- Mentions that their spouse is concerned about their irritability since starting an opioid
- Acknowledges physiological withdrawal symptoms between doses or says, "I swear the tramadol isn't even helping … I just keep taking it to avoid withdrawal."
- Has no prescribed opioid in their urine drug screen
- Tests positive for an alcohol metabolite in the presence of their prescribed opioid
- Tests positive for an illicit drug in the presence of their prescribed opioid
- Forges or alters a prescription

How did you come to your decisions about permissible versus concerning behaviors? Did you base your responses on clinical intuition or experience? Review of known epidemiological risk factors for substance abuse? Knowledge of opioid use disorder (OUD) criteria?

Challenge: How to Navigate Opioid Discussions with Your Patients

The pressure to have discussions about opioid management with your patients can be overwhelming. With recent surveys suggesting that 11 million individuals in the United States—or 3.4% of the population—are using a daily prescription opioid regimen,[1] chances are high that you have encountered these challenges in your practice. Surveys of practicing physicians reveal concern and anxiety about opioid prescribing, with fears ranging from lack of knowledge of which opioids or which doses to use, side effects, and tolerance to diversion or causing addiction (e.g., [2,3]). Such "opioiphobia," if you will, can be a potential barrier to adequate, comprehensive treatment of pain.[4]

The role of long-term opioid therapy for non-cancer pain is not exactly clear-cut. Think about your own personal clinical practice—you may easily be able to conjure up an image of a patient who is doing well with minimal side effects and a good history of compliance, is working full time, and is engaged in their hobbies while on an opioid regimen. You may just as easily identify a patient whose quality of life has been diminished by opioid use or who concerns you with their patterns of medication use.

Over the past 30 years, clinicians have received sometimes urgent and often conflicting messages from various stakeholders about long-term opioid use. The pendulum shift in opioid prescribing guidance has been catalyzed by legal and regulatory events, accumulation of clinical observations, as well as the trajectory and media coverage of epidemiological opioid use/abuse data. You may have felt a push at one point in your career, driven largely by certain dubious pharmaceutical company marketing practices touting the safety and limited addiction potential of long-acting opioids, to eliminate suffering by treating a patient's pain aggressively. For some in-depth analyses of the origins of the "opioid epidemic," please refer to the Further Reading section at the end of this chapter.

Perhaps you then noticed the pushback from some cross-sectional studies that correlated opioid use with negative quality-of-life outcomes and that questioned the long-term benefits of higher-dose opioid regimens.[5–8] At some point, you likely read the briefs and papers from your national academic/scientific pain or family practice organization that took the stance that pain should be considered as a "fifth vital sign"[9] and that opioids are a reasonable option for pain management in carefully selected and monitored patients. Indeed, the 2011 report by the Institute of Medicine[10] and the 2017 revised model policy from the Federation of State Medical Boards[11] have re-affirmed opioids as appropriate for certain patients with chronic non-cancer pain if other first-line non-opioid or non-medication methods have been unsuccessful.

In recent years, you may have felt pressure to stop prescribing opioids altogether regardless of clinical benefit to the individual patient. Like many others, you possibly cited the 2016 guidelines from the U.S. Centers for Disease Control and Prevention (CDC)[12] as a reason for changing your prescribing practices. State medical and pharmacy boards, the media, hospital administrators, state and local governments, insurance funders, and other stakeholders have all weighed in. You may have received threatening letters from pharmacies or third-party payors suggesting that you would be added to a "list of overprescribers" or that you'd be dropped from an insurance panel if you failed to get your patients' MMEs (morphine milligram equivalence) down to some arbitrary number.

Many clinicians have overcorrected and initiated rapid forced tapers due to fear—fear of contributing to the "opioid epidemic," fear of litigation for "overprescribing" consequences, fear of consequences from insurance funders. CDC data show that the total number of annual opioid prescriptions dispensed, after a steady increase starting in 2006, dropped from its 2012 peak (255 million) to 168 million in 2018.[13] On top of getting figurative whiplash from the U-turns of opioid practices, clinicians may start to wonder whom we are here to serve—the patient? The payor? The epidemiologists? The regulatory boards? The community? There is a common "less is better" misperception that reducing opioids is the best option across the board, but we need to keep in mind that new health risks can emerge during an opioid deprescribing experience. This is not necessarily a "risk–benefit" analysis we're confronted by here but rather a "risk–risk" situation: weighing the risk of continuing opioids versus the risk of deprescribing. The seemingly "easier" path is to follow a one-size-fits-all approach to tapering toward an arbitrary MME daily dose target. However, the more accurate (and more difficult) challenge is how to have frank and empathic conversations with your individual patients about their opioid use and to taper the right patient with the right approach at the right time.

Patient Context: The Default Is Pain and Wanting To Be Seen for the "Person Behind the Pain"

Patients also are tasked with weighing the risks and benefits of opioid use, without the training afforded to clinicians. As such, patients tend to interpret potential risks of medications in the context of the more immediate risks of the pain itself. This is evident in comments made to us such as, "I'd trade an earlier death for relief of the pain I have now." A survey study exposed that despite experiencing opioid-related side effects such as constipation or drowsiness, perceived risk of increased pain with decreased opioid medication was more salient.[14] This preference was voiced by patients both with and without opioid tapering experience.

Studies of patient narratives surrounding opioid use underscored similar themes of concern about "forced" dose tapers causing increased pain.[15] Furthermore, patients feel resentful when such tapers are driven not by care for them as a person, but rather solely to meet bureaucratic guidelines that cause them to have to "prove their worth."[16] Step into their shoes for a moment. Imagine you have been humming along with a daily dietary intake of

2,000 calories. Your weight is in a healthy body mass index (BMI) range, you have no major medical diagnoses, and you are moderately active. At your next primary care visit, you're confronted with this conversation:

CLINICIAN: "I see you're eating 2,000 calories per day. You're going to need to cut your calorie intake by 25%."

YOU: "Um, what? Why?"

CLINICIAN: "Due to the obesity crisis in America, the American Medical Association (AMA) recently published new average calorie recommendations. For people of your gender, age, and activity level, they recommend a 1,500-calorie diet."

YOU: "But I'm not obese."

CLINICIAN: "But you are eating food, and the AMA says I have to do this."

YOU: "Is this a law?"

CLINICIAN: "Uh, well, no, it's a guideli-..."

YOU: "But you know me: I choose my food responsibly, and I'm doing my part by exercising and hydrating and..."

CLINICIAN: "Sorry, it's out of my hands. Starting tomorrow you'll be eating a 1,500-calorie diet."

YOU: "What if I'm really hungry or want to eat out at a restaurant or go for a long run?"

CLINICIAN: "Nope. 1,500 calories is as high as you can go."

As you can extrapolate from this tongue-in-cheek example, message framing and consideration for a patient's unique circumstances are important. This isn't a perfect analogy because we need calories to live, but patients who benefit from their opioid regimens may feel that their medication is just as vital for their survival. From a dosing point of view on paper, reducing a client from 120 to 90 MME might hit an arbitrary "target," but this 25% dose reduction—especially if forced all at once by suddenly switching from a 30 mg QID to TID regimen, for example—might make a large impact on a patient's function and quality of life, especially during the dose transition. Also imagine the concern surrounding the "what ifs?"—hunger in the example above, intolerable pain intensity and loss of functional abilities in the case of pain and opioids.

Data from the 2017 National Survey on Drug Abuse[17] revealed that the primary reason given (63% of respondents) for misuse of opioids was to relieve pain, compared to 13% who used opioids to "get high" and vastly outweighing other reasons such as to relieve tension, to improve sleep, to potentiate the effects of other substances. or to experiment. Such results suggest that if we are to attempt to curb opioid misuse though deprescribing or other methods, attention must be paid to giving patients access to better self-management techniques and alternative interventions for pain control.

Interestingly, emerging research[18,19] suggests that when opioids are tapered in a collaborative care model with interdisciplinary support, for the majority of patients the pain either remains stable or decreases slightly. However, some patients do experience increased pain after doses are reduced. So, although it is appropriate to use these data to enhance the willingness of reticent patients to try a gentle opioid taper, we cannot speak in absolutes. Keep your phrasing in mind: say "your pain *may actually* get better" rather than "your pain *will* get better."

Other potential unintended consequences of forced opioid tapers demand attention. Termination of care in response to tapering demands places patients on chronic opioid therapy at risk. A large retrospective cohort study of opioid tapers with a two-year follow-up period found that compared to patients in the sample who were continued on opioids, a 30% opioid taper was associated with greater than four times the odds of termination of care.[20] Consider where your patients may turn for their poorly controlled pain or to ease withdrawal symptoms. They face difficulty finding new providers and may seek illicit sources of opioids.

Another iatrogenic risk possibility with involuntary opioid discontinuation is that of suicidality. There are few large-scale studies investigating suicidal ideation, attempts, or completed suicides as a direct result of opioid deprescribing. Case reports have documented the medical-legal consequences following suicides of patients with chronic pain who were undergoing opioid tapers or were terminated from treatment for aberrant drug behaviors.[21,22] Such cases highlight issues of "standard of care" in opioid tapers and allegations of medical abandonment. A recent retrospective cohort study of patients with chronic pain revealed that discontinuation of chronic opioid therapy as tracked by an "opioid registry" was associated with increased mortality.[23] Most of the deprescribing was initiated by the clinician for a variety of reasons: urine toxicology abnormalities, behavioral issues such as missed appointments or dosing disagreements, or safety concerns such as a mental health condition or past substance use disorder.

For patients whose opioids were discontinued, compared to those who remained on the hospital registry, the hazard ratio was 2.94 for possible or definite overdose death after adjusting for demographic variables.[23] It is unclear using an observational study design whether the high-risk behaviors that led to the opioid discontinuation contributed to the risk of overdose death, if patients sought other means to control their pain, or if some of the overdoses were intentional suicides. In a study of Veterans Health Administration patients following opioid discontinuation, 9.2% had suicidal ideation only while 2.4% had suicidal self-directed violence.[24] Mental health diagnoses such as posttraumatic stress disorder and psychotic disorders were associated with having suicidal thoughts or behaviors in this sample, which suggests that high-risk patients require close monitoring and risk prevention if you do choose to taper or discontinue chronic opioid therapy.

Clinician Context: Cutting Through the Fear and Maintaining a Rational Approach to Opioid Discussions

We Face a Challenging Landscape of Overdose Risk Data and Misapplication of Clinical Guidelines

We cannot ignore the compelling statistics about the trends in opioid overdose deaths in the United States. According to the CDC's WONDER database with complete data through 2018, national drug overdose deaths involving any opioid increased from 1999 to 2017, with the first slight decrease occurring in 2018.[25] Overdose deaths from prescription opioids decreased by 13.5%, while deaths from synthetic narcotics such as fentanyl and fentanyl analogs continued to rise. Not only does the national discussion often neglect to counterbalance opioid overdose statistics with attention to the crisis of uncontrolled chronic pain, the fact that illicit fentanyl and heroin are driving the current opioid overdose epidemic more than prescription opioids gets buried with use of the "opioid crisis" umbrella terminology.[26]

Of course, opioid overdose deaths are just the tip of the iceberg. For every overdose death reported, there are survived overdoses, individuals who develop an iatrogenic OUD, and a percentage who misuse prescription opioids. Studies suggest that approximately 21% to 29% of patients who are prescribed opioids misuse them, with 8% to 12% developing an OUD.[27] Evidence suggests that risks for misuse, overdose, and OUD are associated with higher dose regimens and chronic use.[28-30] However, a recent study examined prevalence of opioid prescription fills and trends in MME prescribed during the 12-month period prior to a diagnosis of OUD or overdose.[31] The authors discovered that that over one-third of patients had an absence of opioid prescription fills in the year before incident OUD or overdose. The implication is that a proportion of patients may have used nonprescription opioids (e.g., illegally obtained pharmaceutical opioids, heroin, or synthetic fentanyl) to achieve pain control or achieve euphoric effects prior to their OUD diagnosis or overdose. Consider a patient who has lost opioid tolerance after a period of reduced opioid exposure—returning to opioid use at previous doses may prove fatal.

In the study just described,[31] among the patients who did have opioid prescriptions in the year preceding OUD diagnosis, the majority were prescribed a mean daily dose below 90 MME. Literature has suggested that the minimum dose for increased risk of opioid overdose is as low as 20 MME,[32] depending on individual genetic differences in metabolism or use of other sedating prescription medications (i.e., polypharmacy risks). A recent study[33] affirmed that sustained discontinuation of chronic opioid therapy was associated with an approximate 50% reduction in risk of overdose but also noted that *dose variability* (e.g., >27.2 MME) was associated with significantly increased risk of overdose compared with low dose variability, independent of total opioid dose. In other words, in well-intentioned attempts to prevent opioid overdose, clinicians may inadvertently be creating conditions that lead to overdose.

Taken together, the data underscore the message that simply relying on definitions of "high doses" versus "low doses" or the current risk stratification algorithms is insufficient to recognize all patients at risk. As mentioned, many have cited the March 2016 CDC Guidelines for Prescribing Opioids for Chronic Pain[12] as the catalyst for driving opioid discontinuation. However, we urge a careful re-reading of those guidelines, which were intended as a voluntary guide—not a mandate, not a law—to address gaps in the knowledge and comfort level of primary care physicians treating patients with opioids. The guidelines proposed a careful and balanced approach. Caution against the use of high-dose opioid analgesics was encouraged, but the authors acknowledged that some patients might still see benefit from opioids, sometimes at high doses, especially those on long-term therapy who developed a physical dependence on the medication. The guidelines have since been used to justify policies that define "maximum" MME doses for all patients regardless of their individual circumstances.

Indeed, as pushback to the drastic change in prescribing habits provoked in part by the publication of the 2016 CDC guidelines and the 2017 frenzy surrounding opioid overdose data, there has been an outcry from various agencies against rapid, forced opioid discontinuation. For example, Human Rights Watch issued a report on the subject in December 2018,[34] stopping short of calling the widespread misapplication of the CDC guidelines a human rights violation. In 2018, the AMA adopted a series of resolutions that called for restraint in implementing the CDC guidelines.[35] In 2019 several former directors of the White House Office of National Drug Control Policy joined health professionals and professional medical organizations in signing a letter to the CDC informally known as the HP3 letter (Health Professionals for Patients in Pain).[36] In response, the U.S. Food and Drug Administration cautioned against abrupt opioid discontinuation,[37] and the CDC itself published a bold clarification on the intent of the guidelines, noting that "policies should allow clinicians to account for each patient's unique circumstances."[38]

You Are Not Alone in Finding These Conversations Difficult

Studies of primary care providers find that chronic pain care is a strong source of frustration, feeling overwhelmed, burnout, and job dissatisfaction. Attitudes are partly based in concerns about the believability of patients' reports of pain and secondary gain[39] but are also influenced by previous experiences with patients who had substance use disorders as well as fear of contributing to physical dependence on opioids.[40] Clinician–patient encounters about opioids can easily shift toward transactions characterized by competition for control,[41] with clinicians giving orders, rejecting patients' ideas or attempting to negotiate, and patients listing reasons or disagreeing.

According to problematic integration (PI) theory as applied to health-related experiences, communication is used to understand and cope with uncertainty. Uncertainties in clinical conversations about opioids tend to center on the amount of information (e.g., about risks and benefits of opioids) and probability judgments (e.g., is this patient misusing, is this patient trustworthy). In a study of Veterans Affairs primary care physicians, uncertainty in opioid discussions was confronted with either offering reassurance, providing education, gathering more information, or avoiding opioids altogether.[42]

We speak of empathy on the part of the clinician being essential to pain care,[43] but clinicians need to adopt self-care strategies to reduce "compassion fatigue" from caring for difficult patients. Developing a set of tools and heuristics to use in conversations with your patients about opioids and opioid tapering can hopefully take some of the guesswork and anxiety out of the process.[44]

Differentiate Between Patients of Concern Due to High-Dose Regimen Versus Identifying Patients with OUD

As mentioned earlier, dosing alone provides a limited picture of opioid risk without considering mental disorders, personal and family histories of substance use, concomitant medication use, and other risk factors. Certainly, involuntary tapering is indicated in certain circumstances, such as after a nonfatal overdose event. One compelling study revealed that in commercially insured patients who had a nonfatal overdose event during long-term opioid therapy for non-cancer pain, opioids were dispensed to 91% of patients within 300 days of an overdose, usually from the same prescribing clinician.[45] At two years, the cumulative incidence of a repeated overdose was 17% for patients receiving high doses of opioids after the initial overdose.

If a one-size-fits-all approach is imprudent, how do we go about determining who is appropriate for an involuntary taper versus who can continue successfully on opioid therapy with proper risk mitigation strategies versus who may be receptive to trying a slow opioid taper using a collaborative care approach. As with suspicion of any disease, the answer comes down to screening for risk factors and clarifying an accurate diagnosis. This step, of course, involves conducting a thorough assessment including interview questions combined with subjective and/or objective testing.

Risk Factors for Misuse, Overuse, or Overdose

Large-scale reviews and analyses have been conducted to elucidate predictors of opioid risk. The two-part series in the 2017 special issue on opioid guidelines in *Pain Physician Journal* provides an excellent updated review of opioid abuse predictors.[46,47] It is important to understand the demographic and psychosocial risk factors and have a method in your clinical practice to screen for comorbid psychopathology, suicidality, and substance use disorders. As mentioned earlier in the chapter, higher-dose regimens and recent dose transitions may pose risks as well.

Let's revisit some of those "yellow/red-flag risks" like we asked you to do in the beginning of this chapter. What's your gut concern when a patient asks for an early refill: overuse or diversion? What if they will be on vacation on the day of their refill and hope to get that task taken care of before they head out of town? When a new patient says, "The only thing that works for me is Roxicodone," how do you know if their specificity is a sign of addiction to that opioid or if they truly have tried all other opioids in their 10-plus years of living with pain and this is where they've landed for best relief? What if a patient declines a lumbar MRI to document pathology or an epidural steroid injection? You may get suspicious of their motives for refusing, but consider that other barriers may exist: the cost of an imaging or procedure copayment, reluctance to endure increased pain from lying flat on the MRI table, lack of transportation to the appointment, severe claustrophobia, or a needle phobia they're too embarrassed to disclose.

Luckily, you don't have to "go it alone" with your risk analysis. To assist with treatment planning, there are several choices of helpful questionnaires; links are provided in the Further Reading section at the end of the chapter. The CAGE-AID[48] is a commonly used instrument consisting of four questions. A single "yes" response renders 79% sensitivity and 77% specificity for identifying problematic substance use behaviors. The Addiction Behaviors Checklist[49] captures a host of aberrant drug behaviors, such as forging or stealing prescriptions, changing the route of administration, deterioration in functioning, concurrent abuse of alcohol or illicit drugs, repeated use of multiple physicians, and so on. The Opioid Risk Tool[50] is also commonly used in addition to interview data. It gives different weights to known risk factors for opioid misuse and suggests low-, moderate-, or high-risk stratification measures. There are different weights for men and women based on research into the risk factors of family or personal history of substance abuse, age between 16 and 45 years, adverse childhood experiences such as preadolescent sexual abuse, and untreated psychological disorders.

Other quality questionnaires or clinician-based interviews have been reviewed and summarized well elsewhere (e.g., [51,52]) and include the SOAPP-R, the COMM, the DIRE, and the Brief Risk Interview. It must be noted that these measures have varying degrees of specificity and sensitivity. No one test has emerged as the gold standard, and results may vary depending on the clinical setting. For example, emerging evidence suggests that these questionnaires, which were developed in the outpatient pain management setting, do not categorize risk well among patients presenting with pain in emergency departments.[53] It is still advised to use a clinical interview combined with PDMP review and a measure of your choosing before beginning opioid treatment, with periodic check-ins throughout long-term opioid therapy. Questionnaire measures should not be used as predictors to deny treatment, but rather as a guide for a treatment plan stratified by risk. For example, an individual in a high-risk category based on remote risk factors could still be treated with opioid management given careful oversight (e.g., more frequent appointments, more frequent urine drug testing, random pill counts, required use of a timed and locked medication dispenser, referral for psychological support).

Addiction Versus OUD

The American Society of Addiction Medicine uses the term *addiction*. Addiction is defined as a primary, chronic disease of brain reward, motivation, memory, and related circuitry and the biopsychosocial manifestations. Addiction is characterized by the "four Cs" as a mnemonic device:

- COMPULSION to use
- Loss of CONTROL of amount or frequency of use
- CRAVING
- Use despite CONSEQUENCES

Like other chronic diseases, addiction often involves cycles of relapse and remission. Without treatment or engagement in recovery activities, addiction is progressive and can result in disability or premature death.

It is important to note that the fifth edition of the American Psychiatric Association's *Diagnostic and Statistical Manual of Mental Disorders*

(DSM-5)[54] no longer uses the terms *substance abuse* and *substance dependence*, and it does not use the term *addiction* as diagnostic. Rather, it refers to categories of "substance use disorders," which are defined along a spectrum of pathology and impairment. Examples include tobacco use disorder or cannabis use disorder. Mild, moderate, or severe specifiers are determined by the number of diagnostic criteria met by the individual.

Table 6.1 lists the DSM-5 criteria for OUD. A cluster of two or three items warrants a "mild" severity specifier (ICD-10-CM F11.10), with four or five items for "moderate" (ICD-10-CM F11.20), and six or more for the "severe" category (also ICD-10-CM F11.20).

Please note the caveat near the bottom of the criteria list that withdrawal and tolerance are signs of physical dependence but do not in and of themselves signify OUD or addiction. To repeat: withdrawal or tolerance alone is not sufficient for a diagnosis of OUD. A patient who worries about an opioid taper does not necessarily meet criteria for OUD. Simply being on a high-dose regimen does not equal OUD.

If you suspect OUD, use this as the opportunity to foster further discussion and offer potentially lifesaving information and interventions. You may recognize that a subset of your patients are in "fuzzy" zones. Perhaps they do not meet criteria for OUD, but they manifest persistent withdrawal symptoms when tapers are attempted; are employing "chemical coping" behaviors to control mood disorders and anxiety with opioids; have untreated mental health conditions; or are not abusing medications themselves but rather are diverting the opioids. Use your best clinical judgment to guide discussions about voluntary opioid tapers or medication-assisted treatment (MAT).

Voluntary Opioid Tapers Versus MAT

The specific nuts and bolts of how to guide dose reductions or opioid discontinuation is beyond the scope of this chapter. We refer the reader to the excellent October 2019 Guide for Clinicians on the Appropriate Dosage Reduction or Discontinuation of Long-Term Opioid Analgesics by the U.S. Health and Human Services Administration (HHS).[55] This document includes a helpful flowchart on determining which patients may be appropriate for deprescribing through a gentle collaborative dose reduction versus which patients may need referral for MAT.

Several community-based programs for voluntary opioid tapering have been tested and show great promise,[19,56] but they do involve patience (e.g.,

Table 6.1 DSM-5 diagnostic criteria for opioid use disorder

A problematic pattern of opioid use leading to clinically significant impairment or distress, as manifested by at least two of the following, occurring within a 12-month period:

Category	Criteria
Impaired control	• Opioids are often taken in larger amounts or over a longer period than was intended. • There is a persistent desire or unsuccessful efforts to cut down or control opioid use. • A great deal of time is spent in activities necessary to obtain the opioid, use the opioid, or recover from its effects. • Craving, or a strong desire or urge to use opioids.
Social impairment	• Recurrent opioid use resulting in a failure to fulfill major role obligations at work, school, or home. • Continued opioid use despite having persistent or recurrent social or interpersonal problems caused or exacerbated by the effects of opioids. • Important social, occupational, or recreational activities are given up or reduced because of opioid use.
Risky use	• Recurrent opioid use in situations in which it is physically hazardous. • Continued opioid use despite knowledge of having a persistent or recurrent physical or psychological problem that is likely to have been caused or exacerbated by the substance.

Physiological/ Pharmacological properties	• *Tolerance, as defined by either:
	  a) a need for markedly increased amounts of opioids to achieve intoxication or desired effect;
	  b) a markedly diminished effect with continued use of the same amount of an opioid.
	• *Withdrawal, as manifested by either:
	  a) the characteristic opioid withdrawal syndrome within minutes to several days after cessation of heavy/prolonged opioid use (e.g., dysphoric mood, nausea or vomiting, muscle aches, lacrimation or rhinorrhea, pupillary dilation, sweating, diarrhea, piloerection, yawning, fever, or insomnia);
	  b) opioids (or a closely related substance) are taken to relieve or avoid withdrawal symptoms.

* This criterion (withdrawal, tolerance) is not considered to be met for those taking opioids solely under appropriate medical supervision.

four to five months of guidance for gradual and flexible MME reductions) and support interventions such as patient education for self-management of pain and/or weekly meetings with a clinician.

MAT is considered the best treatment option for moderate to severe OUD as part of a comprehensive treatment plan. It encompasses use of one of several medications (e.g., buprenorphine, naltrexone, or methadone) in combination with psychosocial and/or behavioral therapy through either office-based programs (e.g., Suboxone programs) or community treatment centers. Buprenorphine can only be prescribed and dispensed by a certified provider who has a Drug Enforcement Agency license and has undergone training to qualify for a Drug Addiction Treatment Act of 2000 waiver. Methadone can only be dispensed through an opioid treatment program that is accredited by an accrediting body approved by the U.S. Substance Abuse and Mental Health Services Administration (SAMHSA). Maintenance therapy with methadone[56] and buprenorphine[57] has been shown to be more effective than control groups receiving no opioid or placebo for treatment of OUD. Unfortunately, institutional and administrative barriers contribute to the underuse of medication for OUD. Not everyone who needs help gets it, so your efforts to connect your patients with local resources is appreciated.

Communication

Conversations about opioid risk and OUD offer prime examples of when it is prudent to avoid the use of "you" judgment statements like "You have a problem," "You're taking too many opioids," and "You are addicted." So, put simply, the first rule of thumb is this: don't start sentences with the word "you." Here are some alternative suggestions on how to open up and foster such discussions. These are not intended to be recited in order. Just use what feels right for you based on the situation.

Build Empathy by Using Reflective Listening and Empathetic Statements

Let patients know you believe and empathize with the severity and impact of their pain. Recognize that most patients are fearful of the pain and potential for dose reduction. You can even express genuine frustration that there is no "quick fix" for their pain.

- *"I understand you have been struggling and I know that discussing pain medicines can be distressing."*
- *"What I hear you saying is that you really want your pain to be reduced."*
- *"So, the opioid doesn't seem to be working as well as it used to."*

Discuss Aberrant Medication-Taking Behaviors in a Nonjudgmental Way

- Use **open-ended questions.** For instance, don't ask *"Are you overusing your oxycodone?"* but rather *"Tell me how you use your oxycodone on a difficult pain day and on a calmer pain day."* Allowing patients to tell the story in their own words helps you listen for positive "change talk," like, "I'd like to take less medicine during flares" or "I've been wondering if there's anything different I can do when I start to feel between-dose withdrawal."
- *"It seems as if you are running out of your medication more quickly than anticipated."*
- *"Sometimes people become too comfortable with the medications and start to take them for reasons other than pain."*

Help Dismantle Unfair Stereotypes by Avoiding Stigmatizing Language

Use language that will not reinforce prejudice or shame.

- **Drug abusers:** This term defines people solely by their behavior around substances. Avoid these labels and instead use person-first language to describe patients or research participants (e.g., "person with a substance/opioid use disorder"). Remember that we don't treat other diseases this way ("Oh, clearly she is a food abuser").
- **Clean/dirty:** These terms are often used to describe urine drug testing results and sometimes the person themselves. Consider using more

cautious language about results, such as "consistent or inconsistent with prescribed regimen."

Take Ownership of the Concern ("I" and "We" Statements)

Although it might seem simpler to "blame the bureaucracy" for dosing decisions, patients deserve your efforts to develop a risk monitoring and mitigation plan rather than using arbitrary dosing targets as a surrogate. Just as patients appreciate a simple acknowledgment if you're running late for their appointment, taking responsibility for the concern about their opioid use can go a long way to foster the therapeutic relationship.

- *"My main goal is to provide care that leads to the healthiest version of 'you' in the long term."*
- *"I want you to have the best possible care, and this difficult but productive conversation is a first step for us."*
- *"I'm becoming concerned about continuing your opioid therapy in these circumstances."*
- *"The medication regimen has become a problem in itself. This is a known complication of therapy that we should not ignore."*
- *"I am concerned about your overuse of opioids and believe you meet the criteria for opioid use disorder, a serious but treatable medical condition."* There is not really a need to split hairs here and mention that OUD is considered a DSM-V *mental* disorder at this point. Keep that door to receptivity open.

Normalize the Problem

- *"All kinds of people can have problems with opioids. You are not alone."*
- *"Getting help for this is like getting help for any other chronic medical problem."*

Address the Concerns or the OUD Diagnosis Head-On and Be Honest

- *"Your behaviors meet the criteria for something known as opioid use disorder. It's helpful to put a name on it because it opens up a variety of approaches to help."*
- *"Continuing the current medication is not a reasonable option due to the risks, but there are options for treating what we call opioid use disorder."*
- *"Opioids have a limited role in management of chronic pain, and before we start you down that path, let's see if we can explore all of the other medical and self-management techniques."* (Declare your whole-person treatment philosophy, and remember that holding back on "new starts" is the best way to decrease opioid prescriptions.)

Explain Treatment Methods Clearly and Let Patients Know They Are Not Alone

- *"There are a number of treatment options. Let's explore them together."*
- *"We will work together to find a treatment plan that works best for you."*
- *"What are your concerns about reducing your opioids?"*
- Given them a "safety net"—discuss non-opioid and non-pharmacologic strategies for coping with pain. See the Further Reading section at the end of the chapter for recommendations on a pain self-management reading list for patients.

Examine the Patient for Signs of Flexibility and Readiness to Taper

You can gauge whether a patient is focused more on obtaining more opioid or on pain relief by asking:

- *"I believe an epidural block and physical therapy can help you. Why don't we wait on any dose increase until after you've completed your PT?"*
- *"Have you given any thought to your long-term course of opioid use?"*

If You Are Guiding a Voluntary Opioid Taper

- *"If I may, I'd like to share with you the health benefits of reducing medications. The intent of this is not to leave you suffering."*
- *"This is not about taking something away from you. It's about treating your pain better with lower risks."*
- *"Research shows that for most patients who gradually reduce their opioid doses, pain either stays the same or actually improves. We also notice that sleep tends to improve with opioid reduction, and that can even further help with pain coping."*
- *"Would you be willing to try a very, very slow dose reduction to see if we can get reductions in your pain? We'll try to go so slow your body won't even realize it. In the meantime, we'll give you other tools to help the areas of your life impacted by pain."*
- *"What would you like your taper to look like?"*
- *"We'll partner together to see each other a bit more frequently during the next few months so I can check in on how this is going for you. Dose decreases will be slow and you'll have the option to pause for a while when needed."* Use the HHS or other tapering guidelines to provide a framework for percentage MME decreases.
- Consider very slow, micro-dose decreases at the start to build the patient's confidence and control. Avoid talk of ultimate dosing targets or "zero" MME.
- *"Let's consider this a trial ... we'll just see how you do and adjust as needed."* This leaves it open-ended if the patient needs to pause or return to previous doses.
- Create a safety plan—let patients know whom they can call if they are having trouble. Assess patients for mood disorders and suicidality, and document accordingly.
- Offer adjuvants for pain management and perhaps even for opioid withdrawal symptoms (e.g., clonidine for autonomic symptoms, nonsteroidal anti-inflammatories [NSAIDs] for myalgias, trazodone for sleep disturbance).
- Offer resources for support:
  - *"Everyone can wean down on opioids, but the trick is to go very slowly and use skills to keep yourself calm as your body adjusts. It might be helpful as we start this process for you to have additional support to*

help with pain and stress. I'd like to give you some names of pain psychologists in the area for you to connect with for the additional coaching."

- If you have space and enough patients going through the process, consider running a weekly or monthly support group.

Be Non-stigmatizing of MAT

Patients with moderate to severe OUD require different care pathways than a voluntary opioid taper. Reassure patients that effective treatments are available:

- *"As we've discussed, your condition meets criteria for moderate opioid use disorder. We find that individuals with that level of impact do best with a treatment that helps to reduce withdrawal symptoms, attends to the cravings, and helps to stabilize brain chemistry. Using a medication to assist your recovery greatly improves your chances of long-term success."*
- *"Nowadays, these programs we call medication-assisted therapy are offered in many different treatment settings, from residential treatment facilities to outpatient programs to even primary care office settings. They involve medications like buprenorphine and methadone. Let's find one that is right for you."*
- *"What the medications—buprenorphine or methadone—do is to make the brain think it's still getting the opioid, but the medicine prevents cravings and withdrawal symptoms and reduces the risk of overdose."*
- Offer referral to specialty addiction treatment. Know how to access MAT programs in your area. Encourage patients to see what is covered by their insurance plan. Often, office-based buprenorphine programs and community methadone clinics are cash-based only, which may be a tangible barrier to patient participation.
- Create a handout for your waiting room or have links on your website where patients can find local MAT programs. See the Further Reading section for treatment locators.
- Reassure patients that you will still offer non-opioid-based suggestions for pain management; you are not abandoning their *pain* care solely to the MAT program.

If You Have to Terminate Therapy Altogether

- Consider a "discharge the molecule, not the patient" approach. You can discontinue a treatment (either through the collaborative approach or through referral to MAT) that has become too risky for the patient without "firing" the patient. Consider the trajectory for the discharged patient—where might they go next without guidance? You can commit to caring for them, but just without a treatment that you feel is no longer helping them.
- If the patient's behavior has been egregiously threatening or disruptive and you decide to terminate them from your practice immediately, make sure you follow your state medical board's recommendations for terminating care (e.g., a letter with explanation, guidance on how to seek other medical care).

References

1. Mojtabai R. National trends in long-term use of prescription opioids. *Pharmacoepidemiol Drug Safty* 2018;27(5):526–534.
2. Lin JJ, Alfandre D, Moore C. Physician attitudes toward opioid prescribing for patients with persistent noncancer pain. *Clin J Pain* 2007;23(9):799–803.
3. Bhamb B, Brown D, Hariharan J, Anderson J, Balousek S, Fleming MF. Survey of select practice behaviors by primary care physicians on the use of opioids for chronic pain. *Curr Med Res Opin* 2006;22(9):1859–1865.
4. Bennett DS, Carr DB. Opiophobia as a barrier to the treatment of pain. *J Pain Palliat Care Pharmacother* 2002;16(1):105–109.
5. Eriksen J, Sjogren P, Bruera E, Ekholm O, Rasmussen NK. Critical issues on opioids in chronic non-cancer pain: an epidemiological study. *Pain* 2006;125(1-2):172–179.
6. Dillie KS, Fleming MF, Mundt MP, French MT. Quality of life associated with daily opioid therapy in a primary care chronic pain sample. *J Am Board Fam Med* 2008;21(2):108–117.
7. Sjogren P, Gronbaek M, Peuckmann V, Ekholm O. A population-based cohort study on chronic pain: the role of opioids. *Clin J Pain* 2010;26:763–769.

8. White JM. Pleasure into pain: the consequences of long-term opioid use. *Addict Behav* 2004;29:1311–1324.

9. American Pain Society Quality of Care Committee. Quality improvement guidelines for the treatment of acute pain and cancer pain. *JAMA* 1995;274:1874–1880.

10. Institute of Medicine (US) Committee on Advancing Pain Research, Care, and Education. *Relieving Pain in America: A Blueprint for Transforming Prevention, Care, Education, and Research.* Washington, DC: National Academies Press, 2011.

11. Federation of State Medical Boards. Guidelines for the chronic use of opioid analgesics, 2017.https://www.fsmb.org/siteassets/advocacy/policies/opioid_guidelines_as_adopted_april-2017_final.pdf

12. Dowell D, Haegerich TM, Chou R. CDC guideline for prescribing opioids for chronic pain—United States, 2016. *MMWR Recomm Rep* 2016;65(No. RR-1):1–49.

13. Center for Disease Control and Prevention. U.S. opioid prescribing rate maps, 2018. https://www.cdc.gov/drugoverdose/maps/rxrate-maps.html

14. Frank JW, Levi C, Matlock DD, Calcaterra SL, Mueller SR, Koester S, Binswanger IA. Patients' perspectives on tapering of chronic opioid therapy: a qualitative study. *Pain Med* 2016;17(10):1838–1847.

15. Huang CJ. On being the "right" kind of chronic pain patient. *Narrat Ing Bioeth* 2018;8(3):239–245.

16. Szalavitz M. No one should have to prove their worth to get medical care, regardless of addiction or pain. *Narrat Inq Bioeth* 2018;8(3):233–237.

17. Han B, Compton WM, Blanco C, Crane E, Lee J, Jones CM. Prescription opioid use, misuse, and use disorders in U.S. adults: 2015 national survey on drug use and health. *Ann Intern Med* 2017;167(5):293–301.

18. Murphy JL, Clark ME, Banou E. Opioid cessation and multidimensional outcomes after interdisciplinary chronic pain treatment. *Clin J Pain* 2013;29(2):109–117.

19. Darnall BD, Ziadni MS, Stieg RL, Mackey IG, Kao M-C, Flood P. Patient-centered prescription opioid tapering in community outpatients with chronic pain. *JAMA Intern Med* 2018;178(5):707–708.

20. Perez HR, Buonora M, Cunningham CO, Moonseong H, Starrels JL. Opioid taper is associated with subsequent termination of care: a retrospective study. *J Gen Intern Med* 2020;35:36–42.

21. Fishbain DA. Medico-legal rounds: medico-legal issues and breaches of "standards of medical care" in opioid tapering for alleged opioid addiction. *Pain Med* 2002;3(2):135–142.

22. Fishbain DA, Lewis JE, Gao J, Cole B, Rosomoff R. Alleged medical abandonment in chronic opioid analgesic therapy: case report. *Pain Med* 2009;10(4):722–729.

23. James JR, Scott JM, Klein JW, Jackson S, McKinney C, Novack M, Chew L, Merrill JO. Mortality after discontinuation of primary care-based chronic opioid therapy for pain: a retrospective cohort study. *J Gen Intern Med* 2019;34(12):2749–2755.

24. Demidenko MI, Dobscha SK, Morasco BJ, Meath THA, Ilgen MA, Lovejoy TI. Suicidal ideation and suicidal self-directed violence following clinician-initiated prescription opioid discontinuation among long-term opioid users. *Gen Hosp Psychiatry* 2017;47:29–35.

25. Centers for Disease Control and Prevention. WONDER. http://wonder.cdc.gov/

26. Rose ME. Are prescription opioids driving the opioid crisis? Assumptions vs. facts. *Pain Med* 2018;19(4):793–807.

27. Vowles KE McEntee ML, Julnes PS, Frohe T, Ney JP, van der Goes DN. Rates of opioid misuse, abuse, and addiction in chronic pain: a systematic review and data synthesis. *Pain* 2015;156(4):569–576.

28. Braden JB, Russo J, Fan MY, Edlund JM, Martin BC, DeVries A, Sullivan MA. Emergency department visits among recipients of chronic opioid therapy. *Arch Inten Med* 2010; 170(16):1425–1432.

29. Sullivan MD, Edlund MJ, Fan MY, DeVries A, Braden JB, Martin BC. Risks for possible and probable opioid misuse among recipients of chronic opioid therapy in commercial and Medicaid insurance plans: the TROUP study. *Pain* 2010;150(2):332–339.

30. Edlund MJ, Martin BC, Russo JE, DeVries A, Braden JB, Sullivan MD. The role of opioid prescription in incident opioid abuse and dependence among individuals with chronic noncancer pain: the role of opioid prescription. *Clin J Pain* 2014;30(7):557–564.

31. Wei YJ, Chen C, Fillingim R, Schmidt SO, Winterstein AG. Trends in prescription opioid use and dose trajectories before opioid use disorder or overdose in US adults from 2006 to 2016: a cross-sectional study. *PLoS Med* 16(11): e1002941. https://doi.org/10.1371/journal.pmed.1002941

32. Adewumi AD, Hollingworth SA, Maravilla JC, Connor JP, Alati R. Prescribed dose of opioids and overdose: a systematic review and meta-analysis of unintentional prescription opioid overdose. *CNS Drugs* 2018;32(2):101–116.

33. Glanz JM, Binswanger IA, Shetterly SM. Association between opioid dose variability and opioid overdose among adults prescribed long-term opioid therapy. *JAMA Network Open* 2019;2(4):e192613. doi:10.1001/jamanetworkopen.2019.2613

34. Human Rights Watch. "Not allowed to be compassionate": chronic pain, the overdose crisis, and unintended harms in the U.S. 2018. https://www.hrw.org/report/2018/12/18/not-allowed-be-compassionate/chronic-pain-overdose-crisis-and-unintended-harms-us

35. American Medical Association. Policy finder: inappropriate use of CDC guidelines for prescribing opioids D-120.932. 2019. https://policysearch.ama-assn.org/policyfinder/detail/CDC%20guideline?uri=%2FAMADoc%2Fdirectives.xml-D-120.932.xml

36. Kertesz SG, Satel SL, DeMicco J, Dart RC, Alford DP. Opioid discontinuation as an institutional mandate: questions and answers on why we wrote to the Centers for Disease Control and Prevention. *Subst Abus* 2019;40(4):466–468.

37. U.S. Food and Drug Administration. FDA identifies harm reported from sudden discontinuation of opioid pain medicines and requires label changes to guide prescribers on gradual, individualized tapering. 2019. https://www.fda.gov/drugs/drug-safety-and-availability/fda-identifies-harm-reported-sudden-discontinuation-opioid-pain-medicines-and-requires-label-changes

38. Dowell D, Haegerich T, Chou R. No shortcuts to safer opioid prescribing. *N Engl J Med* 2019;380:2285–2287.

39. Matthias MS, Parpart AL, Nyland KA, Huffman MA, Stubbs DL, Sargent C, Bair MJ. The patient–provider relationship in chronic pain care: providers' perspectives. *Pain Med* 2010;11:1688–1697.

40. Dobscha SK, Corson K, Flores JA, Tansill EC, Gerrity MS. Veterans affairs primary care clinicians' attitudes toward chronic pain and correlates of opioid prescribing rates. *Pain Med* 2008;9:564–571.

41. Matthias MS, Krebs EE, Collins LA, Bergman AA, Coffing J, Bair MJ. "I'm not abusing or anything": patient-physician communication about opioid treatment in chronic pain. *Patient Educ Couns* 2013;93(2):197–202.

42. Tait RC. Empathy: necessary for effective pain management? *Curr Pain Headache Rep* 2008;12(2):108–112.

43. Eggly S, Tzelepis A. Relational control in difficult physician-patient encounters: negotiating treatment for pain. *J Health Commun* 2001;6(4):323–333.

44. Kennedy LC, Binswanger IA, Mueller SR, Levi C, Matlock DD, Calcaterra SL, Koester S, Frank JW. "Those conversations in my experience don't go well": a

qualitative study of primary care provider experiences tapering long-term opioid medications. *Pain Med* 2018;19(11):2201–2211.

45. Larochelle MR, Liebschutz JM, Zhang F, Ross-Degnan D, Wharam JF. Opioid prescribing after nonfatal overdose and association with repeated overdose: a cohort study. *Ann Intern Med* 2016;164(1):1–9.

46. Kaye AD, Jones MR, Kaye AM, Ripoli JG, Galan V, Beakley BD, Calixto F, Bolden JL, Urman RD, Manchikanti L. Prescription opioid abuse in chronic pain: an updated review of opioid abuse predictors and strategies to curb opioid abuse: part 1. *Pain Physician* 2017;20:S93–S109.

47. Kaye AD, Jones MR, Kaye AM, Ripoli JG, Jones DE, Galan V, Beakley BD, Calixto F, Bolden JL, Urman RD, Manchikanti L. Prescription opioid abuse in chronic pain: an updated review of opioid abuse predictors and strategies to curb opioid abuse: part 2. *Pain Physician* 2017;20:S111–S133.

48. Brown RL, Rounds LA. Conjoint screening questionnaires for alcohol and other drug abuse: criterion validity in a primary care practice. *Wisconsin Med J* 1995;94(3):135–140.

49. Wu SM, Compton P, Bolus R, Schieffer B, Pham Q, Baria A. The Addiction Behaviors Checklist: validation of a new clinician-based measure of inappropriate opioid use in chronic pain. *J Pain Symptom Manage* 2006;32(4):342–351.

50. Webster LR, Webster RM. Prediction aberrant behaviors in opioid-treated patients: preliminary validation of the Opioid Risk Tool. *Pain Med* 2005;6(6):432–442.

51. Jones T, Moore T, Levy JL, Daffron S, Browder JH, Allen L, Passik SD. Comparison of various risk screening methods in predicting discharge from opioid treatment. *Clin J Pain* 2012;28(2):93–100.

52. Ducharme J, Moore S. Opioid use disorder assessment tools and drug screening. *Mo Med* 2019;116(4):318–324.

53. Chalmers CE, Mullinax S, Brennan J, Vilke GM, Oliveto AH, Wilson MP. Screening tools validated in the outpatient pain management setting poorly predict opioid misuse in the emergency department: a pilot study. *J Emerg Med* 2019;56(6):601–610.

54. American Psychiatric Association, *Diagnostic and Statistical Manual of Mental Disorders: Diagnostic and Statistical Manual of Mental Disorders*. 5th ed. Arlington, VA: American Psychiatric Association, 2013.

55. U.S. Department of Health and Human Services. *HHS Guide for Clinicians on the Appropriate Dosage Reduction or Discontinuation of Long-Term Opioid Analgesics*. Washington, DC: US Department of Health and Human Services, 2019.

56. Sullivan MD, Turner JA, DiLodovico C, D'Appollonio A, Stephens K, Chan Y-F. Prescription opioid taper support for outpatients with chronic pain: a randomized controlled trial. *J Pain* 2017;18(3):308–318.

57. Mattick RP, Breen C, Kimber J, Davoli M. Methadone maintenance therapy versus no opioid replacement therapy for opioid dependence. *Cochrane Database Syst Rev* 2009;2009(3):CD002209. doi:10.1002/14651858.CD002209.pub2

58. Mattick RP, Breen C, Kimber J, Davoli M. Buprenorphine maintenance versus placebo or methadone maintenance for opioid dependence. *Cochrane Database Syst Rev* 2014;(2):CD002207. doi:10.1002/14651858.CD002207.pub4

Further Reading

Analysis of the Opioid Crisis

Lembke A. *How Doctors Were Duped, Patients Got Hooked, and Why It's So Hard to Stop.* Baltimore: Johns Hopkins University Press, 2016.

Macy B. Dopesick: *Dealers, Doctors, and the Drug Company That Addicted America.* New York: Little, Brown and Company, 2018.

Quinones S. *Dreamland: The True Tale of America's Opiate Epidemic.* New York: Bloomsbury Press, 2016.

Risk Tools for Download

Addiction Behaviors Checklist: https://www.nhms.org/sites/default/files/Pdfs/Addiction_Behaviors_Checklist-2.pdf

CAGE-AID: http://www.cqaimh.org/pdf/tool_cageaid.pdf

Opioid Risk Tool: https://www.drugabuse.gov/sites/default/files/files/OpioidRiskTool.pdf

Opioid Tapering Guidelines or Resources

Berna C, Kulich RJ, Rathmell J. Tapering long-term opioid therapy in chronic noncancer pain: evidence and recommendations for everyday practice. *Mayo Clin Proc* 2015;90(6):828–842.

U.S. Department of Health and Human Services. *HHS Guide for Clinicians on the Appropriate Dosage Reduction or Discontinuation of Long-Term Opioid Analgesics.* Washington, DC: U.S. Department of Health and Human Services, 2019.

Self-Management/Non-Opioid Tools for Chronic Pain Management

Caudill M, Benson H. *Managing Pain Before It Manages You.* New York: Guilford Press, 2016.

Darnall B. *Less Pain, Fewer Pills: Avoid the Dangers of Prescription Opioids and Gain Control over Chronic Pain.* Boulder, CO: Bull Publishing Company, 2014.

Darnall B. *The Opioid-Free Pain Relief Kit: 10 Simple Steps to Ease Your Pain.* Boulder, CO: Bull Publishing Company, 2016.

Doleys DM. *Understanding and Managing Chronic Pain: A Guide for Patients and Clinicians.* Denver, CP: Outskirts Press, 2014.

Pain Toolkit: https://www.paintoolkit.org/

Peer support website: American Chronic Pain Association (ACPA): www.theacpa.org

Treatment Locators

Methadone Clinic Locator: http://www.opiateaddictionresource.com/treatment/methadone_clinic_directory

National Treatment Referral Helpline: 1-800-662-HELP (4357) or 1-800-487-4889

SAMHSA Behavioral Health Treatment Services Locator (by ZIP code): https://findtreatment.samhsa.gov/treatmentlocator

Suboxone/Buprenorphine Provider Locator: https://buprenorphine.io/find-suboxone-doctor/

Other Resources

CDC 2016 Guidelines: Dowell D, Haegerich TM, Chou R. CDC guideline for prescribing opioids for chronic pain—United States, 2016. *MMWR Recomm Rep* 2016;65(No. RR-1):1–49.

National Institute on Drug Abuse (NIDA) Center of Excellence Opioid Prescribing Resources: https://www.drugabuse.gov/nidamed-medical-health-professionals/opioid-crisis-pain-management/other-opioid-prescribing-resources

Providers Clinical Support System: Offers training and mentors for use of buprenorphine: www.pcssnow.org

SAMHSA: Offers publications such as the Opioid Overdose Toolkit: www.store.samhsa.gov

7

The Depressed/Suicidal Patient

Elizabeth J. Richardson

Case: The Patient Who Feels Helpless and Hopeless in the Face of Their Pain

Perhaps you have had a patient who feels hopeless, dismissing recommendations with a disheartened "Nothing works" and expressing a sense of helplessness to do anything to elevate themselves from their plight. How do you, the clinician, help them overcome these seemingly self-imposed cognitive or emotional barriers to moving forward in their care? What if you hear a patient mention "being a burden" to their spouse, child, or other loved ones or—most concerning—that they would rather not go on living? Patients who communicate such messages can elicit fear and dread from clinicians, since how to further explore these issues with patients and when to refer them to mental health specialists may not seem clear.

Challenge: Understanding Underlying Factors and Scope of Depressive and Suicidal Behavior Among Those with Chronic Pain

A fundamental aspect of human behavior—and most organisms, for that matter—is escape from and avoidance of aversive stimuli. Typically, we first learn to escape a painful situation and then to avoid it, after learning about certain contexts or situations in which that pain could occur again. For example, if you burn yourself pulling something out of the oven, it is highly likely you will pay greater attention on guiding your arm in and out of the oven the next time you cook. Put simply, you learned and now you exert control over the interaction with your environment to avoid that pain.

In the late 1960s, Martin Seligman and Steven Maier discovered a phenomenon that changed how we understand depressive behaviors in the face of painful adversity. In their original work,[1] dogs were harnessed and placed in one of three conditions inside a chamber. Some dogs received escapable shocks, the termination of which was contingent upon the dog's response of pressing a panel, while other dogs received inescapable shocks, with no ability to control the nature and duration of those shocks. A third control group of dogs were simply harnessed in the chamber without receiving any shocks. When the dogs were later placed back in chambers but were not restrained from escaping, something interesting occurred. The control dogs and those that were able to previously control the shock quickly fled to safety. However, the dogs that had been conditioned to expect suffering without a way out passively endured the shock without any effort to escape. Subsequent studies of similar paradigms in humans produce quite similar results. Maier and Seligman[2] even noted that people in lab-based inescapable situations often remarked along the lines of "Nothing worked, so why try?"—quite likely a familiar expression to many health care providers aiming to provide their patients with various treatment modalities for chronic pain. Seligman deemed this behavioral manifestation within the context of perceived uncontrollability *learned helplessness*, and the construct was considered to overlap heavily with symptoms of depression.[3] Pertinent to the *self-efficacy* and *locus of control* concepts introduced earlier in this book, perceiving pain management as improbable or outside of one's control can precipitate or exacerbate passivity, ineffective coping, and depressive symptoms in the face of pain.

While the concept of learned helplessness seems to affirm findings of depression as a potential consequence of chronic pain,[4] there is also evidence that those with depression are at higher risk of developing chronic pain and greater disability from that pain.[5] In other words, the direction of the pain–depression relationship is unclear, but the comorbidity is strong, as approximately half of those with chronic pain exhibit clinically significant depressive symptoms.[6–8] The prevalence of depression appears even higher among those with one of the most common forms of persistent pain—chronic low back pain.[9–11]

Patients with chronic pain and comorbid depression may often be seen as "difficult," a perception that might inadvertently result in negative countertransference from the provider. Patients with both pain and depression fare worse with management of their pain,[12] and the degree to which provider perceptions or other patient-related factors underlie this barrier remains unclear. Nonetheless, depression in the context of chronic pain is concerning, not only for its impact on health and quality of life for the patient, but also because it is a risk factor for suicide.[13]

Among the general population, suicide is the 10th leading cause of death,[14] and alarmingly, there has been a steady increase in the number of suicides nationwide over the past decade.[15] The rate of suicide is higher among those with chronic pain,[16,17] with one review indicating the risk of suicide is double the rate found within the general population.[13] A desire to escape from pain yet feeling hopeless and helpless to do so in daily life has been proposed as a process escalating suicide risk in chronic pain.[13] Others have found that individuals with pain also have changes in the reward circuitry of the brain that may increase susceptibility to suicidal tendencies.[18] It is for these reasons that the presence of chronic pain is considered a common risk factor that clinicians should explore when assessing suicide risk.[19] A large proportion of individuals who die by suicide saw their primary care physician/general practitioner within the few months preceding their death.[20,21] Thus, medical providers are well positioned to assess for depression and suicidality and can serve as a crucial intermediary between the patient and a mental health specialist.

Clinician Context: Knowing How and When to Assess for Depression and Suicidal Ideation

Approaching the patient about depressive symptoms, much less inquiring about suicidal ideation, can be uncomfortable. In fact, primary care physicians explore suicidal ideation in only 36% of patients who present with depressive symptoms, and this percentage is further reduced if patients do not make a direct request about receiving treatment, such as antidepressant therapy, for their symptoms.[22] When the topic is broached, it may often be in the form of a brief, closed-ended question about suicidal ideation (e.g., "Any thoughts of wanting to harm yourself today?") embedded within an intake interview. Such questions may also be asked routinely but in a perfunctory way (e.g., within an electronic medical record checklist) at follow-up visits for patients with known comorbid psychiatric disorders. One problem with this type of question is that it reduces a complex and potentially multifaceted issue to a simple dichotomy. A "no" response by the patient stops the conversation around that issue and may result in an erroneous assumption by the clinician that depression and suicidal ideation can now be moved outside of the scope of clinical focus.[23]

The relatively low proportion of instances in which depression and suicidal ideation are explored with patients may be due to fear about what will occur. Below are some common thoughts that can occur with the prospect of evaluating a patient for suicidal ideation:

"If I ask about suicidal ideation, the patient will get offended." Actually, research shows that when physicians ask their patients about suicidal ideation, patients more highly rate the care they receive from that physician.[24] More importantly, addressing suicide risk and ideation with patients was predictive of remission of patients' depressive symptoms six months later.[24] Exploring suicidality is patient-centered and may serve to demonstrate the provider's concern for the patient and therefore deepen the therapeutic alliance.

> *"If I mention suicide, they may now think of it as an option."* A common myth is that introducing the topic of suicide poses an iatrogenic risk. In other words, asking about suicide may cause the patient to more deeply reflect on thoughts of self-harm and act on those thoughts, particularly among high-risk patients. However, research has consistently demonstrated that asking about suicidal ideation is not associated with increases in suicidal ideation.[25,26]

> *"If I ask whether they are suicidal, what if they say yes?"* Here, the reasons for the clinician's apprehension can be twofold.

> > First, the clinician may not feel confident in their ability to effectively navigate a further risk assessment and triage if the patient endorses suicidal ideation. The unfortunate consequence is that the provider may avoid the topic altogether or instinctively ask about suicidal ideation in a manner that elicits a negative response. For example, asking the patient "You're not feeling suicidal, are you?" may send

the message that "no" is the correct answer and that you may not be open to any other answer.[27] Additionally, responding with words like "good" to a negative answer by a patient can also reinforce the notion that it is a topic off-limits within the patient–clinician relationship.[27]

Second, the clinician may anticipate a costly digression from an already time-constrained schedule to work on the problem and identify the best mode of care for a patient who endorses suicidal ideation. This concern more likely stems from apprehension of "the unknown" and low self-competence in handling a positive depression and/or suicidal screen, should it occur. Primary care physicians are typically well versed in triage of physical symptoms and navigation of differential diagnoses, and suicide risk assessment operates much the same way. Indeed, primary care providers who felt more competent about handling suicidal ideation were more willing to explore this issue with patients.[28] By learning more about the risk factors, effective ways to assess for depression and suicidality, and extending the patient's care via mental health referrals, you will gain more comfort in addressing these issues with your patients.

Effectively Evaluating Depression and Suicide in the Context of Chronic Pain

Identifying whether suicidal ideation is present is a crucial first step.[23,29] Questions should be worded in a manner that allows the patient to respond more freely, without assuming implicit constraints imposed by the provider. For example, framing the question in a supportive way (e.g., "Some people can feel at the end of their rope, and that their pain has made life no longer worth living. Have you felt this way?")[27] may (1) normalize such feelings within the patient, thus lessening the patient's apprehension of expressing them, and (2) couch the question in an empathic way, thus improving the therapeutic alliance.

If a patient endorses suicidal ideation, recommendations for continued assessment range from a stepwise method of questioning the patient[29,30] to the use of more elaborate algorithms for risk stratification.[19] In the stepwise method, if suicidal ideation is present, the physician should then take steps to better understand the nature of the patient's suicidal thoughts. Distinction can be made between passive or active suicidal ideation among those with chronic pain, with the former being somewhat more commonly reported.[31] Passive suicidal ideation is often characterized as feeling one would be better off dead but without a specific plan or intent to do so. Phrases such as "I wish I just wasn't here" or "Some days I wish I just wouldn't wake up" are often indicative of a passive desire for escape or death. Active ideation, on the other hand, typically entails thoughts about how the individual might act on that desire, such as, "I've thought about just finishing off the bottle of medication" or "I've thought about taking my gun and ending it all." Active ideation is typically seen as more urgent in the hierarchy, although this does not mean the physician should dismiss any passive ideation that is present. A passive desire for death may serve as a precursor to more definitive forms of suicidality[32] and thus presents a prime opportunity for early intervention.

The clinician should next ask if the patient has a *plan* to act on those thoughts, and if so, if there is *intent* to carry the plan out. Patient endorsement of items further along this hierarchy can indicate greater imminent risk and the need for more urgent management.[19] A critical aspect of assessing a patient's suicide plan and intent is whether or not they have access to the means they would use to carry out a suicide plan. Similar to the broader population, the majority of those who had chronic pain and who died by suicide did so by use of a firearm (53.6%).[33] Yet, discussion of the availability of a firearm and gun safety is infrequent among primary care providers.[34] Clinicians may anticipate that discussion of limiting gun access may be a potentially polarizing topic, and the provider may fear that any recommendations for doing so would be met with resistance, thereby damaging the patient–provider relationship.[35] Interestingly, though, most patients report that discussion about firearms with providers is needed and should occur,[35] suggesting that this fear is somewhat unwarranted. Even so, framing questions about access to firearms within an empathic context can help maintain the therapeutic alliance in the cases where such a discussion may prove difficult.

Use of motivational interviewing strategies (see Chapter 2) can also increase the likelihood that the patient will adopt recommendations for safe storage of firearms. Storage recommendations may include use of trigger locks, keeping firearms in a locked cabinet and giving the key to family members or loved ones, or temporarily relocating firearms outside the home.[36]

Intentional overdose on opioids is another means of suicide among those with chronic pain.[33] Therefore, clinicians should also assess patients' access to any opioid medications outside the purview of the provider. This may include asking about leftover medications from any prior prescriptions or whether others in the home are regularly taking prescription opioids. Opioid dosing recommendations,[37] frequency of urine screens and follow-up monitoring,[38] and availability of medication-assisted therapy[39] may mitigate the risk for suicide or unintentional overdose, but these are somewhat outside of the scope of this chapter. Nevertheless, clinicians are encouraged to review this literature.

In-Office Screens for Depression and Suicidal Ideation

Some patients may be more inclined to disclose depression and/or suicidal ideation on a self-report measure than in a face-to-face interview.[40] There are several self-report tools that assess both the degree of depressive symptoms and the presence of suicidal ideation; however, the Patient Health Questionnaire-9 (PHQ-9)[41] was developed specifically for use with patients in primary care settings.[42] The PHQ-9 is brief and easy to administer, with only nine items to reflect *Diagnostic and Statistical Manual of Mental Disorders* (DSM) symptoms of major depressive disorder. Higher scores on the PHQ-9 are indicative more severe depressive symptoms, with a cutoff score of 10 indicating a high likelihood for the presence of major depression [43]. The PHQ-9 is freely available along with other PHQ modules, including generalized anxiety disorder-7 (GAD-7). Consideration should be given to also exploring anxiety with patients, given that anxiety in the context of chronic pain has also been associated with increased suicide risk.[44]

Over the last 2 weeks, how often have been bothered by any of the following problems? (Use "✓" to indicate your answers)	Not at all	Several days	More than half the days	Nearly every day
1. Little interest or pleasure in doing things	0	1	2	3
2. Feeling down, depressed, or hopeless	0	1	2	3
3. Troubles falling or staying asleep, or sleeping too much	0	1	2	3
4. Feeling tired or having little energy	0	1	2	3
5. Poor appetite or overeating	0	1	2	3
6. Feeling bad about yourself â€" or that you are a failure or have let yourself or your family down	0	1	2	3
7. Trouble concentrating on things, such as reading the newspaper or watching television	0	1	2	3
8. Moving or speaking so slowly that other people could have noticed? Or the opposite â€" being so fidget or restless that you have been moving around a lot more than usual	0	1	2	3
9. Thoughts that you would be better off dead or of hurting yourself in some way	0	1	2	3
FOR OFFICE CODING __0__+____+____+____ =Total score:____				

If you checked off any problems, how difficulty have these problems made it for you to do your work, take care of thing at home, or get along with other people?			
Not different at all	somewhat difficult	Very difficult	Extremely difficult
☐	☐	☐	☐

Developed by Drs. Robert L. Spitzer, Janet B.W. Williams. Kurt Krownke and colleagues, with an educational grant from Pfizer Inc. No permission required to reproduce, translate, display or distribute.

The patient Health Questionnaire -9 (PHQ-9) screen for depression. The PHQ-9 and others, such as screens for generalized anxiety, are free to use and can be downloaded from www.phqscreeners.com

The last item of the PHQ-9 is often used as an initial screen for a patient's suicide risk, and prior research has found a patient's endorsement on this item to be a strong predictor of subsequent suicidal behaviors. Two large studies found that outpatients who endorsed item 9 on the PHQ-9 were at higher risk of suicide attempt and death within the following year;[45] this finding was seen across all age groups.[46] It should be noted that no screening or self-report measure on its own is adequate in assessing risk.[19] We recommend that the clinician always review results of the PHQ-9 (or any other screen) with the patient during the face-to-face interview, using the stepwise method of evaluating suicidality in an empathic manner.

Implementing an Organized Method of Handling the Suicidal Patient in the Office

What if screening is positive and further questioning by the provider reveals that the patient has a suicide plan, an expressed intent to carry that plan out, poor social support, and access to lethal means, such as firearms? This most serious constellation of factors is undoubtedly every clinician's fear. Established clinical practice guidelines[19] suggest that in these high-risk situations, hospitalization is warranted to maintain the safety of the patient. If the primary care physician has admitting privileges, this will facilitate appropriate transition of care of the suicidal patient, though it is imperative that someone accompany the patient to the hospital, such as a family member if available. If a family member is not available or the provider does not have admitting privileges, emergency 911 personnel can be contacted to transfer the patient to a local emergency department. If the patient refuses, involuntary hospitalization may be an option, depending on the applicable laws of the state in which the provider practices.[47] While the transfer process is under way, it is important to keep the patient in a clinic location where there is no immediate access to any means of self-harm (sharps, cords, tubing or sheets/blankets that can be tied) and the patient should be accompanied by a staff member for observation.[47] Should a high-risk patient like this leave the office against medical advice, local authorities should be immediately notified.

Having an established protocol for patients in crisis can reduce any uncertainty and apprehension about how to handle such situations as well as reduce ambiguity about providers' action steps in caring for those with moderate to low risk of suicide. Moreover, it can also be used as a prevention strategy, particularly for patients who have experienced suicidal crisis events in their history. For example, implementing a safety plan is a recommended action for individuals with chronic pain, limited coping skills, and ongoing psychosocial stressors who may be at risk for becoming acutely suicidal in the future.[19] A safety plan results from a collaborative process between the patient and the provider, with a mutually agreed-upon list of positive coping strategies that the patient agrees to use should a suicidal crisis arise. The safety plan includes a list of warning signs (cues that signal when the patient should implement the plan), coping strategies and social contacts (what the patient can do and who they have identified to call in the event they feel suicidal), their mental health providers or urgent care services that are nearby, and strategies to limit any lethal means, such as having family or friends store firearms.[47] A basic resource that is often provided is a local crisis line (if available) or the National Suicide Prevention Lifeline (1-800-273-TALK). A safety plan template for providers and other patient risk assessment management tools are freely available through the Suicide Prevention Resource Center.[47] Using a standard template allows you to document safety planning with the patient; give patients a hard copy to refer to when they leave your office. While this may take a few moments of your time, you may very well be providing that patient with life-saving tools.

Developing a clinic-wide strategy for handling patients at risk for suicide is also crucial. When clinic staff are all on the same page about what to do in crisis situations, care for the patient is most efficient and effective. Office protocols that identify the nearest emergency department, transportation options, and contact information for mental health providers who may assist with psychiatric admission can minimize interruption of clinic activity.[47] Providers are encouraged to review and use resources available within the Suicide Prevention Toolkit for Primary Care Practices (available at www.sprc.org), which offers strategies and other templates to assist with the development of individualized office protocols and ways to obtain patient education tools that can be supplied by your clinic.

Patient Context: Patient-Specific Factors That Increase Vulnerability to Depression and Suicidal Ideation

Since some patients may not disclose that they are experiencing suicidal thoughts, it is important for the clinician to be aware of certain patient characteristics that may increase vulnerability to depression or suicidal ideation in the context of chronic pain. Even if a patient's symptoms do not currently meet criteria for a depressive disorder or suicidal ideation is truly absent, understanding points of susceptibility will allow you to have a more discerning approach throughout the trajectory of the patient–clinician relationship. This will allow for a more acute awareness of when to implement various treatment modalities or to refer when the need arises.

Patient risk factors for depression and suicidal ideation can be understood as those that are modifiable versus those that are relatively static, with the implication that addressing the former can reduce a patient's depressive symptoms and lessen their overall risk of suicidality.

Static Factors

Risk factors that are not amenable to change by a provider typically include sociodemographic characteristics (e.g., past history, gender, socioeconomic or work status) and type of chronic pain experienced. The prevalence of depression is typically higher in women in both the general population[48] and among those with chronic pain.[49] However, among the general population, White men are at increased risk of death by suicide; other risk factors are being younger, being divorced, having experienced childhood adversities, having made a suicide attempt in the past, or having had a loved one die by suicide.[50] On the other hand, suicidal ideation and attempts, but not completions, appear higher in women.[51]

There are some differences with the general population when considering similar risk factors among those with chronic pain. For example, the gender and age gaps are not as wide among those with chronic pain who die by suicide versus those who do not have chronic pain.[19] Similarly, the association between gender, marital status, or education level and suicidal ideation and/or attempts among those with chronic pain has been less conclusive,[52] although being unemployed or disabled due to the pain condition appears to increase suicide risk.[53] Other pain-specific factors that may increase suicide risk include sleep problems, having multiple forms of pain, frequency of intermittent pain, and negative pain-related cognitions.[52] Experiencing negative pain-related beliefs appears to be predictive of suicidal ideation above and beyond the more static factors,[54,55] and it is encouraging that such maladaptive beliefs are quite modifiable with psychological treatment.

Modifiable Factors

When patients experience significant interference from pain with activities, they may perceive themselves as no longer able to fulfill their established roles in their family, work settings, or other social contexts. Often, family roles may shift in terms of responsibilities, at times even dramatically so, particularly in cases where there is high solicitousness from a spouse or other family members. Coupled with negative thought patterns, such as catastrophizing, this can lead to a perception of being a burden to others. It is not uncommon for individuals with chronic pain to feel as if their limitations impose burden, yet this perception is associated with depression as well as various forms of suicidality.[54] Wilson and others[55] found that one's perception of being a burden in the context of chronic pain was a strong predictor of suicidal ideation, above and beyond functional limitations, pain intensity, and depression. Therefore, a patient's communication to the clinician that contains elements of self-devaluation or self-perceived burden should immediately prompt the physician to assess for depression and suicidal ideation.

A patient's severity of depression and catastrophic thinking about pain are also robust predictors of suicidal ideation, even above patient demographics or characteristics of their pain, such as pain severity and duration.[56] Similarly, the degree to which a patient feels helpless in controlling their pain—a component of pain catastrophizing[57]—is also significantly associated with suicidality.[53] Maladaptive coping strategies, such as catastrophizing, are quite responsive to cognitive-behavioral therapy for chronic pain.[58] Addressing these negative pain-related beliefs will allow the patient to perhaps cope more effectively with the risk factors that are less amenable to change (e.g., upbringing, socioeconomic status, marital status, type of pain diagnosis).

Communication: Relaying to the Patient That Learning Tools to Cope with the Challenges of Chronic Pain Are Within Reach

We opened this chapter discussing Seligman's[3] concept of learned helplessness and its role in depressive behaviors. In the half-century since this concept was introduced, additional behavioral and brain imaging data have been amassed. Maier and Seligman[2] have since suggested that their original theory turned out to be somewhat reversed: passivity in the context of adversity is not what is learned; rather, one *learns* effective strategies to mitigate aversive circumstances to adapt and thrive. In other words, individuals with pain who experience depression or feelings of helplessness or who see no other option in life can acquire the necessary tools to better cope with the challenges of persistent chronic pain.

Less research has been done to understand patient-related factors associated with resilience among those with chronic pain who have experienced significant depression or suicidal ideation. In a community sample of individuals with chronic pain, those who reported they had someone to talk to about important life decisions had higher odds of recovery from suicidal ideation.[58] Further, levels of optimism, a sense of purpose in life, and pain acceptance contribute to psychological resilience in those with chronic pain[59]—factors that can be strengthened through acceptance and commitment therapy.[60]

When and How to Refer a Patient to a Mental Health Specialist

Providing care to the patient with chronic pain is most effective when it is collaborative, with discipline-specific points of intervention requiring cooperation from multiple professionals. Psychologists and other mental health specialists are no exception, given their expertise with addressing the affective and cognitive components contributing to the experience of pain. Therefore, it is rare to prematurely refer someone who has pain in a chronic state, has failed conservative management, or who may be experiencing emotional distress. We suggest referring the patient to a mental health clinician sooner rather than later as part of a comprehensive pain management program, even if it is to solely develop behavioral strategies that may reduce physical limitations from pain (e.g., activity pacing).

As mentioned in the introduction to this book, psychologists and other licensed psychotherapists near your practice can be found via state board of examiners in psychology or counseling. While we highlight the benefit of connecting with pain psychologists, we recognize situations in which these specialists may not be readily available. Referral to any qualified mental health professional is foremost when depression and/or suicidal ideation is a concern. While pain may be a contributing factor to a patient's crisis, there are many other modifiable factors that mental health generalists can effectively address. Clinicians are encouraged to be proactive in connecting and networking with local mental health providers who are in community private practice or who are embedded within larger academic institutions or hospitals. Having their business cards or other referral material on hand for clinic staff and patients can facilitate the referral process.

A patient may initially be resistant to a referral for psychological intervention. Patients may conclude that you perceive their pain to be "all in their head" or that somehow their physical complaints are not being taken seriously. This assumption on the patient's part stems from a very dualistic view that issues are either physical or psychological, with little understanding that they can be both. It is often helpful to reinforce that interventions are not "either/or" but "complementary" in order to tackle the stranglehold pain can have on one's life. Patients may also similarly assume that they are being told that psychological issues are perceived to *cause* their pain complaints, rather than vice versa. Reinforcing the notion that experiencing pain on a daily basis can deplete one's ability to cope with life stressors can validate their physical complaints while also normalizing the emotional distress that co-occurs. A helpful analogy that is used by some pain psychologists is to present the pain experience as the result of an equation that includes both what is physically felt and the emotions that are experienced:

Pain = Physical Sensations + Emotional Distress

This analogy is consistent with research showing separate neural pathways that encode the negative affective valence of pain.[62] However, when viewed in this simple way, patients can understand how their pain can be changed by targeting nociception (what the patient understands as the physical sensation of pain), typically the aim of the medical providers. Patients can also see how their emotional or psychological state can influence the resulting pain experience.[63] As an example for patients, let's suppose that an individual accidentally smashed his thumb while doing some repair work. Leading up to and surrounding the accident, we might consider two scenarios. In one scenario, the individual received a reprimand by his supervisor, got into an argument with his spouse, and is reminded of the stack of unpaid bills on his kitchen table. In another scenario, the individual is financially caught up, happened to spend a wonderful day with his spouse, and is up for a promotion at work. In which scenario would the person experience pain more intensely? Most would identify the former situation as more painful and may even recall past personal experiences to this effect. Obviously with chronic pain, the contribution of emotional distress is more complex, as the presence of depression can more substantially impact the pain experience as well as reduce one's ability to cope with fleeting frustrations encountered in life.

In summary, depression is a common comorbidity in chronic pain, and individuals who experience chronic pain are at increased risk of suicide. Primary care clinicians are in a crucial position to assess depression and evaluate for suicidal ideation within this population and to connect individuals with a psychologist or other mental health provider to provide more comprehensive care. Proactively connecting with pain psychologists and other mental health providers in your area will streamline the referral process when the need arises. Developing clinic protocols to assess patients' risk and implementation of safety measures can reduce ambiguity, lessen clinician anxiety, and maintain effective clinic flow while ensuring delivery of quality care for the patient. While patients may initially be resistant to a referral to a mental health provider, framing the benefits of psychotherapy in a way that validates their physical pain while also emphasizing the real emotional distress that co-occurs can improve their openness to psychotherapy. The overall message that can be relayed by the clinician to the patient is one of hope, in that relief from the emotional distress of pain is certainly within reach.

References

1. Seligman MEP, Maier SF. Failure to escape traumatic shock. *J Exp Psychol* 1967;74:1–9.
2. Maier SF, Seligman MEP. Learned helplessness at fifty: insights from neuroscience. *Psychol Rev* 2016;123(4):349–367.
3. Seligman MEP. Learned helplessness. *Ann Rev Med* 1972;23:407–412.
4. Fishbain DA, Cutler R, Rosomoff HL, Rosomoff RS. Chronic pain-associated depression: antecedent or consequence of chronic pain? A review. *Clin J Pain* 1997;13(2):116–137.
5. Young Casey C, Greenberg MA, Nicassio PM, Harpin RE, Hubbard D. Transition from acute to chronic pain and disability: a model including cognitive, affective, and trauma factors. *Pain* 2008;134(1-2):69–79.
6. Fishbain DA, Goldberg M, Meagher BR, Steele R, Rosomoff H. Male and female chronic pain patients categorized by DSM-III psychiatric criteria. *Pain* 1986;26:181–197.

7. Romano JM, Turner JA. Chronic pain and depression; does the evidence support a relationship? *Psychol Bull* 1985;97:18–34.

8. Turk DC, Okifuji A, Scharff L. Chronic pain and depression: role of perceived impact and perceived control in different age cohorts. *Pain* 1995;61:93–101.

9. Krishnan K, France R, Pelton S, McCann S. Chronic pain and depression: 1. Classification of depression in chronic low back patients. *Pain* 1985;22:279–287.

10. Gallagher RM, Moore P, Chernoff I. The reliability of depression diagnosis in chronic low back pain. *Gen Hosp Psychiat* 1995;17:399–413.

11. Richardson EJ, Ness TJ, Doleys DM, Baños JH, Cianfrini L, Richards JS. Depressive symptoms and pain evaluations among persons with chronic pain: catastrophizing, but not pain acceptance, shows significant effects. *Pain* 2009;147:147–152.

12. Bair MJ, Robinson RL, Katon W, Kroenke K. Depression and pain comorbidity—a literature review. *Arch Intern Med* 2003;163(20):2433–2445.

13. Tang NK, Crane C. Suicidality in chronic pain: a review of the prevalence, risk factors and psychological links. *Psychol Med* 2006;36(5):575–586.

14. Kochanek K, Murphy S, Xu J, Arias E. *Mortality in the United States, 2016.* NCHS data brief no. 293. Hyattsville, MD: US Department of Health and Human Services, CDC, National Center for Health Statistics, 2017.

15. Stone DM, Simon TR, Fowler KA, Kegler SR, Yuan K, Holland KM, Ivey-Stephenson AZ, Crosby AE. Vital signs: trends in state suicide rates—United States, 1999–2016 and circumstances contributing to suicide—27 states, 2015. *MMWR Morb Mortal Wkly Rep* 2018;67:617–624.

16. Fishbain DA, Lewis JE, Gao J. The pain suicidality association: a narrative review. *Pain Med* 2014;15:1835–1849.

17. Calati R, Laglaoui Bakhiyi C, Artero S, Ilgen M, Courtet P. The impact of physical pain on suicidal thoughts and behaviors: meta-analyses. *J Psychiatr Res* 2015;71:16–32.

18. Elman I, Borsook D, Volkow ND. Pain and suicidality: insights from reward and addiction neuroscience. *Prog Neurobiol* 2013;109:1–27.

19. Sall J, Breener L, Millikan Bell AM, Colston MJ. Assessment and management of patients at risk for suicide: Synopsis of the 2019 U.S. Department of Veterans Affairs and U.S. Department of Defense clinical practice guidelines. *Ann Intern Med* 2019;171(5):343–353.

20. Luoma JB, Martin CE, Pearson JL. Contact with mental health and primary care providers before suicide: a review of the evidence. *Am J Psychiatry* 2002;159:909–916.

21. De Leo D, Draper BM, Snowdon J, Kõlves K. Contacts with health professionals before suicide: missed opportunities for prevention? *Compr Psychiatry* 2013;54(7):1117–1123.

22. Feldman MD, Franks P, Duberstein PR, Vannoy S, Epstein R, Kravitz RL. Let's not talk about it: suicide inquiry in primary care. *Ann Fam Med* 2007;5(5):412–418.

23. Silverman MM, Berman AL. Suicide risk assessment and risk formulation, part I: a focus on suicide ideation in assessing suicide risk. *Suicide Life Threat Behav* 2014;44(4):420–431.

24. Rossom RC, Solberg LI, Vazquez-Benitez G, Lauren Crain AL, Beck A, Whitebird R, Glasgow RE. The effects of patient-centered depression care on patient satisfaction and depression remission. *Fam Pract* 2016;33(6):649–655.

25. Mathias CW, Furr RM, Sheftall AH, Kapturczak N, Crum P, Dougherty DM. What's the harm in asking about suicidal ideation? *Suicide Life Threat Behav* 2012;42(3):341–351.

26. DeCou CR, Schumann ME. On the iatrogenic risk of assessing suicidality: a meta-analysis. *Suicide Life Threat Behav* 2018;48(5):531–543.

27. Vannoy SD, Fancher T, Meltvedt C, Unützer J, Duberstein P, Kravitz RL. Suicide inquiry in primary care: creating context, inquiring, and following up. *Ann Fam Med* 2010;8(1):33–39.

28. Graham RD, Rudd MD, Bryan CJ. Primary care providers' views regarding assessing and treating suicidal patients. *Suicide Life Threat Behav* 2011;41(6):614–623.

29. McDowell AK, Lineberry TW, Bostwick JM. Practical suicide-risk management for the busy primary care physician. *Mayo Clin Proc* 2011;86(8):792–800.

30. Shea SC. The chronological assessment of suicide events: a practical interviewing strategy for the elicitation of suicidal ideation. *J Clin Psychiatry* 1998;59(suppl 20):58–72.

31. Smith MT, Edwards RR, Robinson RC, Dworkin RH. Suicidal ideation, plans, and attempts in chronic pain patients: factors associated with increased risk. *Pain* 2004;111(1-2):201–208.

32. Baca-Garcia E, Perez-Rodriguez MM, Oquendo MA, Keyes KM, Hasin DS, Grant BF, Blanco C. Estimating risk for suicide attempt: are we asking the right questions? Passive suicidal ideation as a marker for suicidal behavior. *J Affect Disord* 2011;134(1-3):327–332.

33. Petrosky E, Harpaz R, Fowler KA, Bohm MK, Helmick CG, Yuan K, Betz CJ. Chronic pain among suicide decedents, 2003 to 2014: findings from the National Violent Death Reporting System. *Ann Intern Med* 2018;169(7):448–455.

34. Dobscha SK, Denneson LM, Kovas AE, Corson K, Helmer DA, Bair MJ. Primary care clinician responses to positive suicidal ideation risk assessments in veterans of Iraq and Afghanistan. *Gen Hosp Psychiatry* 2014;36:310–317.

35. Walters H, Kulkarni M, Forman J, Roeder K, Travis J, Valenstein M. Feasibility and acceptability of interventions to delay gun access in VA mental health settings. *Gen Hosp Psychiatry* 2012;34:692–698.

36. Runyan CW, Becker A, Brandspigel S, Barber C, Trudeau A, Novins D. Lethal means counseling for parents of youth seeking emergency care for suicidality. *West J Emerg Med* 2016;17(1):8–14.

37. Dowell D1, Haegerich TM1, Chou R1. CDC guideline for prescribing opioids for chronic pain—United States, 2016. *JAMA* 2016;315(15):1624–1645.

38. Im JJ, Shacter RD, Oliva EM, Henderson PT, Paik MC, Trafton JA. Association of care practices with suicide attempts in US veterans prescribed opioid medications for chronic pain management. *J Gen Intern Med* 2015;30(7):979–991.

39. Ma J, Bao YP, Wang RJ, Su MF, Liu MX, Li JQ, Degenhardt L, Farrell M, Blow FC, Ilgen M, Shi J, Lu L. Effects of medication-assisted treatment on mortality among opioids users: a systematic review and meta-analysis. *Mol Psychiatry* 2019;24(12):1868–1883.

40. Yigletu H, Tucker S, Harris M, Hatlevig J. Assessing suicide ideation: comparing self-report versus clinician report. *J Am Psychiatr Nurses Assoc* 2004;10(1):9–15.

41. Spitzer RL, Kroenke K, Williams J. Validation and utility of a self-report version of the PRIME-MD: the PHQ primary care study. Primary care evaluation of mental disorders. Patient health questionnaire. *JAMA* 1999;282:1737–1744.

42. Spitzer RL, Williams JBW, Kroenke K, Linzer M, deGruy FV, Hahn SR, Brody D, Johnson JG. Utility of a new procedure for diagnosing mental disorders in primary care: the PRIME-MD 1000 study. *JAMA* 1994;272:1749–1756.

43. Kroenke K, Spitzer RL, Williams JB. The PHQ-9: validity of a brief depression severity measure. J Gen Intern Med 2001;16:606–613.

44. Sommer JL, Blaney C, El-Gabalawy R. A population-based examination of suicidality in comorbid generalized anxiety disorder and chronic pain. *J Affect Disord* 2019;257:562–567.

45. Simon GE, Rutter CM, Peterson D, Oliver M, Whiteside U, Operskalski B, Ludman EJ. Do PHQ depression questionnaires completed during outpatient visits predict subsequent suicide attempt or suicide death? *Psychiatr Serv* 2013;64(12):1195–1202.

46. Rossom RC, Colman KJ, Ahmedani BK, Beck A, Johnson E, Oliver M, Simon GE. Suicidal ideation reported on the PHQ9 and risk of suicidal behavior across age groups. *J Affect Disord* 2017;215:77–84.

47. Western Interstate Commission for Higher Education Mental Health Program (WICHE MHP) & Suicide Prevention Resource Center (SPRC). *Suicide Prevention Toolkit for Primary Care Practices: A Guide for Primary Care Providers and Medical Practice Managers*. Rev. ed. Boulder, CO: WICHE MHP & SPRC, 2017.

48. Parker G, Brotchie H. Gender differences in depression. *Int Rev Psychiatry* 2010;22(5):429–436.

49. Fishbain DA, Goldberg M, Meagher BR, Steele R, Rosomoff H. Male and female chronic pain patients categorized by DSM-III psychiatric diagnostic criteria. *Pain* 1986;26(2):181–197.

50. Hawton K, van Heeringen K. Suicide. *Lancet* 2009;373(9672):1372.

51. Nock MK, Borges G, Bromet EJ, Cha CB, Kessler RC, Lee S. Suicide and suicidal behavior. *Epidemiol Rev* 2008;30(1):133–154.

52. Racine M. Chronic pain and suicide risk: a comprehensive review. *Progr Neuropsychopharmacol Biol Psychiatry* 2018;87:269–280.

53. Racine M, Choinière M, Nielson WR. Predictors of suicidal ideation in chronic pain patients: an exploratory study. *Clin J Pain* 2014;30(5):371–378.

54. Fishbain DA, Bruns D, Bruns A, Gao J, Lewis JE, Meyer LJ, Disorbio JM. The perception of being a burden in acute and chronic pain patients is associated with affirmation of different types of suicidality. *Pain Med* 2016;17:530–538.

55. Wilson KG, Heenan A, Kowal J, Henderson PR, McWilliams LA, Castillo D. Testing the interpersonal theory of suicide in chronic pain. *Clin J Pain* 2017;33(8):699–706.

56. Edwards RR, Smith MT, Kudel I, Haythornthwaite J. Pain-related catastrophizing as a risk factor for suicidal ideation in chronic pain. *Pain* 2006;126:272–279.

57. Sullivan MJL, Bishop SR, Pivik J. The Pain Catastrophizing Scale: development and validation. *Psychol Assess* 1995;7:524–532.

58. Morley S, Eccleston C, Williams A. Systematic review and meta-analysis of randomized controlled trials of cognitive behaviour therapy and behaviour therapy for chronic pain in adults, excluding headache. *Pain* 1999;80(1-2):1–13.

59. Fuller-Thomson E, Kotchapaw LD. Remission from suicidal ideation among those in chronic pain: what factors are associated with resilience? *J Pain* 2019;20:1048–1056.

60. Sturgeon JA, Zautra AJ. Resilience: a new paradigm for adaptation to chronic pain. *Curr Pain Headache Rep* 2010;14(2):105–112.

61. Hayes SC, Luoma JB, Bond FW, Masuda A, Lillis J. Acceptance and commitment therapy: model, processes and outcomes. *Behav Res Ther* 2006;44(1):1–25.

62. Corder G, Ahanonu B, Grewe BF, Wang D, Mark J. Schnitzer MJ, Scherrer G. An amygdalar neural ensemble that encodes the unpleasantness of pain. *Science* 2019;363:276–281.

63. Bushnell MC, Čeko M, Low LA. Cognitive and emotional control of pain and its disruption in chronic pain. *Nat Rev Neurosci* 2013;14:502–511.

Further Reading

Pain and Depression

Bair MJ, Robinson RL, Katon W, Kroenke K. Depression and pain comorbidity: a literature review. *Arch Intern Med* 2003;163(20):2433–2445.

IsHak WW, Wen RY, Naghdechi L, Vanle B, Dang J, Knosp M, Dascal J, Marcia L, Gohar Y, Eskander L, Yadegar J, Hanna S, Sadek A, Aguilar-Hernandez L, Danovitch I, Louy C. Pain and depression: a systematic review. *Harvard Rev Psychiatry* 2018;26(6):352–363.

Pain and Suicidality

Racine M. Chronic pain and suicide risk: a comprehensive review. *Progr Neuropsychopharmacol Biol Psychiatry* 2018;87:269–280.

Assessing Suicidality

McDowell AK, Lineberry TW, Bostwick JM. Practical suicidal-risk management for the busy primary care physician. *Mayo Clin Proc* 2011;86(8):792–800.

Western Interstate Commission for Higher Education Mental Health Program (WICHE MHP) & Suicide Prevention Resource Center (SPRC). *Suicide Prevention Toolkit for Primary Care Practices: A Guide for Primary Care Providers and Medical Practice Managers.* Rev. ed. Boulder, CO: WICHE MHP & SPRC, 2017.

8

The Anxious Patient

Leanne R. Cianfrini

Case: The Anxious Patient

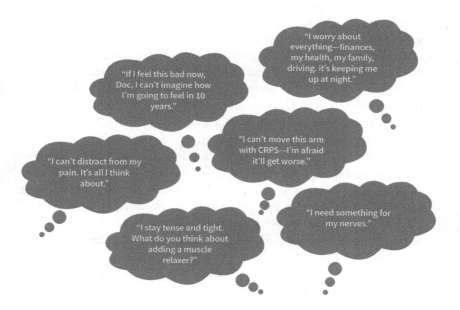

Challenge: Staying Aware of "Normal" Pain-Related Anxiety, Maladaptive Fear of Pain and Movement, and Comorbid Clinical Anxiety Disorders

To some degree, worry about the impact of pain-related functional limitations is normal. Who wouldn't have concern over a change in finances or job stability, increased time and cost for medical appointments, or medical procedures with uncertain risks and outcomes? Even patients with a healthy acceptance of their chronic symptoms may still worry about uncontrolled or unpredictable pain flare days. We know that humans prefer certainty to uncertainty in both experimental studies[1] and in real-life contexts, with variance in the degree to which uncertainty is tolerated.[2] Consider the degree of uncertainty involved in living with a persistent pain condition: potential for diagnostic ambiguity, uncontrollability of the timing and length of flares, a lack of firm guarantees with interventional outcomes, a lack of clarity in risk–benefit analysis for chronic opioid therapy, unclear trajectories for pain intensity and pain impact as one ages. Can you really look a patient straight in the eye and state, "This treatment will eliminate your pain"?

Some fears are adaptive in the short run, as an emotional reaction to specific, identifiable, and immediate threats. Fear may protect an individual from imminent danger (e.g., an injury) as it prompts the "fight-or-flight response" of defensive or protective behaviors. However, in the context of chronic pain, such escape behaviors can actually strengthen fear over time because they prevent individuals from engaging in behaviors that disconfirm their fear belief.

In contrast to fear, anxiety is a future-oriented affective state with a fuzzier and more elusive focus. We also recognize that abnormal anxiety can exist both prior to and after onset of chronic pain (e.g., clinical diagnoses such as generalized anxiety disorder [GAD], panic disorder, or posttraumatic stress disorder [PTSD]). We should be sensitive to the impact of symptoms like intrusive thought ruminations and hypervigilance (scanning for potential sources of threat) as well as physiologic arousal and tension. These cognitive, behavioral, and physiologic symptoms can cause insomnia and fatigue, lead to unhealthy coping strategies, and enhance pain intensity, among other consequences.

Patient Context: "I Just Don't Know How to Turn My Brain Off!"

Anxiety Disorders

An estimated 40 million individuals in the United States (or 18.1% of the population) age 18 and older experience some form of an anxiety disorder every year.[3] Anxiety disorders are a group of conditions sharing features of excessive fear and anticipation of future threat, experienced to a degree that interferes significantly with one's normal routine, occupational or academic functioning, or social activities or relationships, or there is marked distress about having the symptoms. There are several anxiety disorder diagnoses categorized in the fifth edition of the American Psychiatric Association's *Diagnostic and Statistical Manual of Mental Disorders* (DSM-5),[4] summarized in Table 8.1.

PTSD, although related to anxiety and anticipatory fear, is no longer classified under the umbrella of anxiety disorders in the DSM-5. PTSD is triggered by experiencing or witnessing a traumatic event. Symptoms may include flashbacks, nightmares, uncontrolled intrusive thoughts and memories about the event, hyperarousal (easy startle reactivity), insomnia, difficulty concentrating, feelings of detachment, and negative changes in thinking and mood. The individual may exhibit efforts to avoid memories of the distressing event.

Somatic symptom disorder (SSD) is another DSM-5 diagnosis you may encounter in clinical practice. It is not included in the anxiety disorders, but is characterized by the following:

- Somatic symptoms that are distressing or result in significant functional disruption
- Excessive thoughts, feelings, or behaviors related to the somatic symptoms associated with disproportionate and persistent thoughts about the seriousness of the symptoms, persistently high level of anxiety about health or symptoms, and excessive time and energy devoted to these symptoms or health concerns.

The specifier of SSD with "predominant pain" is for individuals whose somatic complaints primarily involve pain. SSD replaced three diagnoses—pain disorder, undifferentiated somatoform disorder, and somatization

Table 8.1 Summary of DSM-5 anxiety disorders

Anxiety Disorder	General Description
Generalized anxiety disorder (GAD)	Excessive anxiety and worry (apprehensive expectation) about a number of events or activities across several domains. The anxiety and worry are associated with symptoms such as restlessness, fatigue, difficulty concentrating, irritability, muscle tension, and/or sleep disturbance.
Specific phobias	Marked and persistent fear, recognized by the individual as excessive or unreasonable, cued by the presence or anticipation of a specific object or situation (e.g., flying, animals, heights). Exposure to the phobic stimulus almost invariably provokes an immediate anxiety response, which leads to avoidance or endurance with intense distress.
Social anxiety disorder	Marked fear or anxiety about one or more social situations in which the individual is exposed to possible scrutiny by others, e.g., social interactions like conversations, being observed eating or drinking, or performing in front of others. The individual fears that he or she will act in a way or show anxiety symptoms that will be negatively evaluated (e.g., humiliation or embarrassment, will lead to rejection or offend others).
Panic disorder	Recurrent, unexpected panic attacks (defined as an abrupt and discrete period of intense fear or discomfort with symptoms such as tachycardia, sweating, trembling, dyspnea, chest discomfort, nausea, dizziness, fear of dying or losing control, etc.). At least one of the attacks is followed by at least a month of persistent concern about having additional panic attacks, worry about the implications or consequences of a panic attack, or a significant change in behavior related to the attacks. This may be diagnosed in the presence or absence of agoraphobia.
Agoraphobia	Marked fear or anxiety about 2 or more of the following situations: using public transport, being in open spaces, being in enclosed places, standing in line or being in a crowd, being outside of the home alone. The individual fears or avoids these situations, and the fear is out of proportion to the actual danger posed by the situation and to the sociocultural context.

disorder—that were included in previous versions of the DSM. The SSD diagnosis is fairly controversial, with critics suggesting that there is a high probability of misdiagnosing chronic pain as a mental illness,[5] which still carries an unfortunate degree of stigma that medical illnesses do not. There is a screening questionnaire, the SSD-12,[6] that operationalizes the DSM-5 criteria if you are interested in a tool for your practice, but it is recommended to be judicious with your use of this diagnosis.

Some unique phobic anxiety scenarios may present themselves in individuals with chronic pain and interfere with treatment. For example, a specific phobia of confined spaces (claustrophobia) might preclude the patient from obtaining a magnetic resonance imaging scan; a meta-analysis showed that 1.2% of people have a claustrophobic event that terminates such a scan.[7] Claustrophobia also affects short-term and long-term adherence to a continuous positive-airway pressure (CPAP) regimen for obstructive sleep apnea.[8] A specific phobia of needles (trypanophobia) might lead a patient to refuse epidural blocks, cortisone joint injections, infusion therapies, electrodiagnostic studies, or acupuncture. Some clients may be embarrassed to bring up their anxiety and risk being judged simply as noncompliant if they refuse diagnostic studies or certain interventions. We will next discuss the impact of another specific fear—the fear of pain itself.

The Fear-Avoidance Model

The fear-avoidance model explains a cyclical pattern of fearful thoughts and avoidance behaviors that self-perpetuates and can lead to negative outcomes. It was developed to explain how a minority of individuals with acute pain following an injury or surgery might transition over time to a chronic state of disability, low mood, and inactivity.[9-11] See Figure 8.1 for a diagram of the essential elements of the original model.

Individuals who have minimal fear of pain (e.g., "it's part of life," "it's part of normal aging," "it's a challenge I can get through") are likely to persist with active coping that confronts pain with movement, continue to engage in meaningful activities, return to work, and often go on to a reasonable functional recovery after injury. However, other individuals may instead interpret pain as an imminent, persistent threat to their well-being and engage in the maladaptive appraisal style of catastrophizing. We presented in

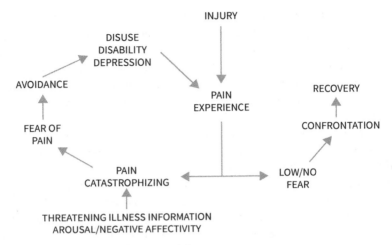

Figure 8.1 The fear-avoidance model
Adapted from reference 11.

Chapter 3 the three factors involved in pain catastrophizing—rumination (a relative inability to inhibit pain-related thoughts in anticipation of, during, or following a painful encounter), magnification (a heightened fear of the threat of pain), and helplessness in the context of pain. This fear of persistent or additional pain can affect attentional processes. We have all seen patients who struggle to distract their attention from pain and seem hypervigilant to even minor fluctuations in physiologic symptoms.

Negative affectivity is a stable disposition to experience a variety of negative emotional states and encompasses a range of constructs including trait anxiety, neuroticism, and pessimism (i.e., a glass half-empty perspective).[12] Threatening illness information may be as simple as "When I tried this stretch, my legs felt a bit numb" or "My surgeon told me if I twist my torso too fast, I could become paralyzed." Both negative affectivity and threatening illness information can fuel catastrophic thinking about pain.

This fear can lead to avoidance behaviors—"I can't work because it will cause more pain," "I'm reluctant to do the physical therapy exercises because they may hurt me more"—followed by disuse, musculoskeletal deconditioning, disability, and depressed mood. Those factors, in turn, lower pain tolerance, lead to overestimation of future pain from activity, and perpetuate the cycle with fewer and fewer attempts to overcome limitations. This model is supported by research showing that high pain-related fear is associated with hypervigilance and unwillingness to engage in activity.[13] Clearly, high pain severity or intensity is in itself a threatening experience that drives escape and avoidance behaviors and has its own role in explaining disability, but the fear of pain and/or re-injury is often a better predictor of disability than pain itself or other biomedical variables.[14,15] The model has been updated over time,[16] and it continues to evolve to incorporate contexts of personal goals, self-regulation, and motivation.[17] There is even functional magnetic resonance imaging (fMRI) evidence to suggest that fear of pain and fear of negative implications of physical symptoms are associated with brain regions such as the medial prefrontal cortex.[18]

Several measures are used to assess fear-avoidance beliefs, and if you notice that one of your patients is particularly guarded and reluctant to move, expresses fear of movement or re-injury ("I'm scared I'm going to re-injure my shoulder"), declines to participate in physical therapy, and/or is disengaging from meaningful activities, it might be helpful to administer one of the following in addition to a depression screener. Assessment is recommended because referrals for psychological intervention may be most appropriate for patients who are more likely to avoid activity. For a critical review and comparison of the psychometric properties of these measures, see the review by Lundberg and colleagues.[19]

Tampa Scale of Kinesiophobia (TSK): This seems to be the most studied measure related to fear avoidance.[11] Kinesiophobia refers to an irrational, devastating fear of movement and activity stemming from the belief of fragility and susceptibility to injury.[20]

Pain Anxiety Symptoms Scale (PASS): This 20-item scale is designed to measure pain-related anxiety in cognitive, physiologic, and motor response domains, and offers clinical interpretation through cutoff scores.[21] Associations have been made between PASS scores and catastrophic thinking.

Fear-Avoidance Beliefs Questionnaire (FABQ): This questionnaire is oriented more toward the fear-avoidance beliefs of individuals who are currently working or who have recently been off work due to pain.[22]

Fear-Avoidance Components Scale (FACS): The newest of the measures, this 20-item scale was designed to be more comprehensive, with items reflecting the various cognitive-behavioral components of the fear-avoidance model, with clear score cutoff points that can be useful for clinicians.[23]

Subclassifications of patients with problematic fear-avoidance beliefs have been proposed.[24] Differences in presentation and belief systems may manifest in patients who are afraid because they are misinformed versus those who have learned to avoid pain based on past experience versus those who avoid due to high levels of distress. For example, a patient who has been told by a clinician that pain always indicates harm and that their spine is vulnerable or fragile ("You have the spine of a 90-year-old!") may be hypervigilant but willing to try painful activities in a limited way. Treatment may involve basic psychoeducation about anatomy and the nervous system, and can include gradual exposure to exercises that restore confidence in the spine or affected body part. In contrast, an "affective avoider" may base their beliefs on a distorted significance of pain (e.g., catastrophizing); such a patient would warrant a more intensive cognitive therapy approach to address the emotionally charged beliefs.

Interestingly, studies have shown that clinicians themselves are moderately fear avoidant,[25] independent of expertise and with remarkable consistency across medical disciplines. This unintentional bias may affect the recommendations we provide.[26] Reflect for a moment on your own personal beliefs about pain and how they may shape your clinical interactions. Are you more likely to prescribe bed rest or exercise? How quick are you to write up return-to-work restrictions? Do you use terminology consistent with a biomedical perspective, like "eliminate" or "cure" the pain, or do you favor more holistic terminology like "manage" or "tame" the pain?

Nonpathological Worry Can Affect Pain and Health as Well

Although the pathological form of worry is a central feature of GAD, nonpathological worry can still affect chronic pain. Early characterizations of worry described the process as "an attempt to engage in mental problem solving on an issue whose outcome is uncertain but contains the possibility of one or more negative outcomes.[27] Worry is common and is essentially a normal process—we've all experienced the "what if?" time-traveling brain, and it can actually convey benefit by maintaining vigilance to the unresolved threat and engaging us in problem-solving strategies.[28] Eccleston and colleagues described the relationship between worry and chronic pain and posited a model of chronic pain in the context of misdirected problem-solving.[29]

To generate empathy for the "stressed" or "stressed-out" patient, take a trip down memory lane back to your medical, nursing, or graduate school training and visualize those index-card study notes on "stress" as a state of threatened homeostasis and Hans Selye's general adaptation syndrome.[30] Recall those diagrams of sympathetic ("fight/flight/freeze") versus parasympathetic ("rest and digest") activity and the role of the hypothalamic–pituitary–adrenal (HPA) axis. Hannibal and Bishop summarized the impact of dysregulated sympathetic adrenergic catecholamines and neuroendocrine hormones such as cortisol on inflammatory processes and pain.[31] We direct interested readers to thorough reviews of corticolimbic connectivity and genetic polymorphisms that modulate the stress response.[32,33]

Clinician Context: The Anxious Patient Poses a Risk for Increased Pain, Opioid Misuse, and Synergistic Sedative/Polypharmacy Burden

Consider the Links Between Anxiety and Pain

Anxiety and chronic pain frequently co-occur. Incidence estimates vary, but one study found that 45% of a sample of primary care patients with chronic musculoskeletal pain screened positive for at least one anxiety disorder[34] and that scores on a variety of pain, function, and other health-related quality-of-life measures worsened as the number of comorbid anxiety disorders increased. Other studies have found that 20% of individuals with chronic low back pain had co-occurring GAD,[35] whereas 40% of a population presenting for interventional pain management procedures screened positive for GAD (compared to 14% of a nonpatient control group).[36] When patients are seen for assessment of chronic pain resulting from a traumatic event such as workplace injuries, burns, or motor vehicle accidents, the prevalence of PTSD is high, with estimates typically ranging from 30% to 50%.[37–39] Two large-scale studies[40,41] found that all of the anxiety disorders (with the exception of agoraphobia without panic disorder) were more likely to occur in individuals with neck and/or low back pain than in people without chronic pain. The highest odds ratios were found for GAD and PTSD.

Compared to patients without anxiety disorders, anxious patients have significantly worse outcomes across multiple pain, pain-related functional interference, psychological, and other health-related quality-of-life measures. Anxiety can also impact response to treatments. PTSD and generalized anxiety have been associated with higher rates of spinal cord stimulation failure leading to explantation.[42] In a study of outcomes from a major interdisciplinary pain rehabilitation program, although patients with chronic pain and anxiety responded with improved functioning following the program, their outcomes were poorer than program participants who didn't have an anxiety disorder.[43] One can understand that the chronic arousal and attentional vigilance associated with anxiety disorders may drain a patient's energy and resources, lowering their motivation to participate in rehabilitation and adhere to treatment regimens.

Furthermore, when depression and anxiety coexist, which they often do, pain is more severe and the comorbidities cause greater interference with daily activities, a higher number of disability days, increased health care utilization, and reduced health-related quality of life.[44,45] An interesting longitudinal "chicken or the egg" study indicated that in patients with chronic pain treated at an outpatient pain specialty clinic, combined symptoms of depression and anxiety predicted future pain intensity and pain-related disability, but the pain variables did not conversely predict prospective mood changes.[46]

Theoretical models and mechanisms have been proposed to explain the high comorbidity between chronic pain and the anxiety disorders.[47] Two of note are the following:

- "Shared vulnerability"—Genetically influenced individual difference factors (e.g., low threshold for alarm or sympathetic dysregulation, high injury sensitivity) predispose individuals to develop anxiety and chronic pain when exposed to certain environmental conditions (e.g., a traumatic incident or physical injury).
- "Mutual maintenance"—Physiologic, emotional, and behavioral components of anxiety maintain or exacerbate pain symptoms and vice versa through pathways such as trauma reminders, attentional and

reasoning biases, or limited use of adaptive strategies due to cognitive demand from symptoms.

Finally, neuroimaging gives us insight into brain regions related to the affective aspects of pain, such as altered fear and emotional processing in the amygdala.[48]

Consider the Link Between Anxiety and Opioid Misuse

Research has demonstrated that mental disorder diagnoses are associated with both an increased likelihood of prescription drug misuse and substance use disorders in general[49–51] and nonmedical use of prescription opioids in particular.[52,53] It has been found that among patients who were prescribed opioids for chronic pain, those who were classified in a high psychiatric morbidity group were significantly younger, had been taking opioids longer, had higher opioid risk testing scores suggestive of aberrant drug behaviors, and had a greater frequency of abnormal urine toxicology screens compared to those who were classified in the low psychiatric morbidity group.[54] A cross-sectional analysis found that 50% of patients with chronic pain who screened positive for generalized anxiety also screened positive for opioid misuse compared to 10% in patients without anxiety.[55]

A longitudinal study sought to address the temporal sequence of mood/anxiety disorders and opioid use disorder—in other words, do preexisting psychiatric disorders lead to nonmedical opioid use or are mood/anxiety disorders a consequence of nonmedical prescription opioid use?[56] Unsurprisingly, evidence was found for multiple pathways:

1. Precipitation of anxiety disorders in patients with baseline nonmedical opioid use and no prior history of psychopathology (consistent with previous findings, e.g., [57])
2. Increased risk of developing OUD among patients with baseline mood disorders
3. A shared vulnerability for nonmedical prescription opioid use and mood/anxiety disorders based on genetic or environmental risks.

So, research suggests that using opioids might initiate development of anxiety disorders. This highlights the importance of screening for and addressing anxiety when treating a patient with chronic pain on opioid therapy. It is also evident that individuals with mood and anxiety disorders might use opioids nonmedically to alleviate their mood symptoms (i.e., "self-medicating").

Consider the Link Between Anxiety, Pain, and Polypharmacy Risks

Although prescription anxiolytics seem like the quickest solution to ease a patient's anxiety, co-prescribing opioids and benzodiazepines brings its own set of challenges and risks. Benzodiazepines ("benzos"), including diazepam, alprazolam, and clonazepam, among others, increase the level of the inhibitory neurotransmitter GABA. The synergistic opioid–benzodiazepine sedative burden can lead to unintentional overdose through respiratory depression.

Across multiple studies of individuals who are prescribed opioids for chronic pain, those receiving a concomitant benzodiazepine had increased risks of experiencing adverse outcomes, including drug-related poisoning, with evidence of a dose–response effect.[58-60] For example, in a cohort study in North Carolina, the overdose death rate among patients who were prescribed both an opioid and a benzodiazepine was 10 times higher than among those receiving only chronic opioid therapy.[61] Guidelines strongly discourage co-prescribing,[62] and many clinicians have instituted policies that opioid therapy will not be started in the presence of a prescription for a benzodiazepine, and vice versa.

Patients often request a muscle relaxant or bedtime sedative–hypnotic as treatment for anxiety. Use your own clinical judgment, keeping in mind sedative risks and perhaps using these requests as a cue to further explore the patient's symptoms and current coping skills repertoire. For example, if worry is keeping a patient up at night, this is a cue to ask about their sleep hygiene and suggest use of cognitive or behavioral coping skills (e.g., a daytime "worry period" with a mindfulness technique at bedtime) rather than jumping immediately into offering a prescription sleep medicine. If a patient's primary complaint is tension or tight muscles from stress, a deep breathing or progressive muscle relaxation technique may be worth a try before adding a sedating muscle relaxer to their regimen. When necessary, non-benzodiazepine medication options for treating anxiety could include a selective serotonin reuptake inhibitor (SSRI; e.g., paroxetine) or a serotonin-norepinephrine reuptake inhibitor (SNRI; e.g., duloxetine). Some medical providers use hydroxyzine or beta-blockers (e.g., atenolol) off-label for treatment of anxiety, but again, caution is used regarding sedative risks when co-prescribing with opioids.

Communication: "Keep Calm and Carry On"

First, take the pressure off yourself. You don't suddenly have to turn into a pain psychologist to be helpful to your patient with stress, fear, or anxiety. If recognition of symptoms and a reasonable mood screen is as far as you can take it, those are great steps toward making the appropriate referrals or self-management recommendations. Guidance on how to make referrals to community psychologists is provided in Chapter 7.

Effective nonmedication treatment of anxiety disorders or even nonpathological "stress" or "worry" in patients with chronic pain is typically done by counselors or psychologists using cognitive–behavioral therapy (CBT) and/or acceptance and commitment therapy (ACT) techniques. If you have a general familiarity with these treatments, you can better explain their usefulness and increase the possibility that the patient will follow through with the recommended referral. See Chapter 2 for a general review of these evidence-based psychotherapeutic modalities. These are self-management approaches that fit with the paradigm emphasizing the role of patients as active and accountable participants in their own health care.

A therapist working with a fear-avoidant patient, for example, may use CBT to address unrealistic fears, test probabilities of the feared worst-case scenarios, reframe catastrophizing beliefs, and confront avoidance behaviors. The patient may be asked to design a fear hierarchy, ranking movements and activities from least feared to most feared for that individual. Through covert imaginal rehearsal of the movements and then in vivo exposure to them, the patient gradually works up the hierarchy to test their movement limits and shift perceived "danger zone" activities back to their "comfort zone." This can be done even more effectively in conjunction with the patient's physical therapist, as graded exposure to exercise and psychoeducation can be provided by a non-psychologist.[63]

ACT can also help patients find a path back to a life with more meaning. ACT in a patient with pain and anxiety may focus on exploring their values (e.g., I have a strong work ethic, I want to be remembered as being a loyal friend) and enhancing motivation to pursue activities consistent with their most cherished values.

Mindfulness-based stress reduction (MBSR) is another promising intervention. Originally developed by Kabat-Zinn,[64] MBSR is a group-based intervention that uses mindfulness exercises at its core to increase awareness of thoughts, sensations, and emotions. Strategies for self-regulation are taught to promote healthy and adaptive responses to stress. Mindfulness can help individuals with chronic pain facilitate the grieving of losses associated with chronic pain (e.g., financial stability, social interaction, spontaneity, ease of movement, ability to plan) and improve acceptance. Mindfulness meditation has been tentatively associated with neuroendocrine and immunological changes, such as reductions in circulating levels of C-reactive protein, that may mediate the benefits for chronic pain.[65,66]

Exercise can also have anxiolytic effects, although it's a bit more of a "hard sell" for patients with chronic pain. If the patient's pain or pathology limits participation in vigorous or high-impact exercises, resistance training, yoga, and tai chi have been found to be reasonably effective alternatives.[67]

In addition to referring for psychotherapy or physical therapy/gym programs, you can become a "talented amateur" (to borrow a phrase from Doug Gourlay, MD) by using some basic techniques to calm in-office interactions when patients present with anxiety so that they will be more receptive to the information you are sharing about their diagnosis or treatment options.

What Not to Say

- *"Well, stop worrying about it!"*
- *"Just relax"* or *"Calm down."* To quote an internet meme: "Never in the history of calming down has anyone ever calmed down by being told to calm down."

- *"Oh no! Degenerative disc disease is really terrible! You better stop moving or it'll get much worse."* Be careful not to inadvertently feed catastrophic thought patterns, give misinformation about the severity of a condition, or promote too much bed rest.

General Suggestions

- **Create a calming environment in your waiting room.**
  - Although distraction is used in multiple forms as a therapeutic technique in settings like pediatric dentistry, benefits for chronic pain and anxiety disorders in adults are usually short-lived. Distraction can actually be characterized as a mental escape/avoidance behavior.
  - A clinic or hospital waiting room can be a hotbed of anticipatory anxiety. Patients may feel impatient or in a rush, may be uncomfortable with pain, may be ruminating on what's about to happen in the appointment, or may feel worried about hygiene as they hear every cough or sniffle from the other patients around them. Anxiety can make wait times feel even longer.
  - However, a clean waiting room with fresh plants, soft music, distraction with neutral or lighthearted television programming at a quiet volume, and/or ambient lighting can temporarily calm nervous patients. Remember that patients with migraines and trauma histories may be affected by strong scents, bright lights, and loud noises.
  - Consider upgrading your reading material. Disorganized magazines strewn about can look chaotic. You can offer a neat display of handouts for relaxation resources. Most people bring their smartphones or tablets, but ask them kindly to limit phone conversations and turn off audio for their games.
  - For patients with chronic pain and anxiety, varied seating can also be a welcome relief. Consider a choice of chairs with arms (for ease of standing), without arms (for larger patients), and chairs positioned near a table (for completing paperwork instead of uncomfortably holding a clipboard or tablet).
- **Include anxiety screening measures as part of your intake questionnaire packet and at periodic follow-ups.**

- You can use your choice of fear-avoidance belief questionnaires mentioned earlier in the chapter if your patient population seems particularly tentative about movement and exercise.
- A valid and efficient screening tool for the presence and severity of GAD is the GAD-7.[68]
- **Have some tools handy in your office.**
  - Consider keeping your anatomical spine or joint model close by, ready to help you illustrate a patient's symptoms. Don't assume that all patients know what a disc looks like, what a "bulge" is versus a herniation, or the difference between the spinal cord and peripheral nerves. Simple education in clear terms with these visual cues can help to de-threaten diagnoses.
  - Find a good diagram of a cross-section of the brain with pain and limbic system structures circled or colored in. This can help you explain how brain circuitry can be impacted by pain or anxiety, and these brain areas can be used as a guide to choose the most effective technique (e.g., *"This is the amygdala. We know this through brain imaging studies to be a region that is activated as a fear center. When it's activated, pain can feel worse and we might want to avoid activity. We also know that certain techniques, like relaxation and mindfulness, can calm down the activation in the amygdala."*).
  - Keep your own phone, smartwatch, or office tablet stocked with a breathing pacer app in case you need to guide a patient through a panic attack.
  - Have a nice "sleep hygiene tips" handout to give to patients with pain- or anxiety-related insomnia. These are easily found online.
- **Be sensitive to possible phobias.** If a patient is hesitating to have a procedure or test done, you can ask directly, *"I notice that you've canceled the nerve conduction study three times now. Tell me a bit about what's happening there—is it a matter of time, cost, or perhaps you're not a fan of needles?"*
- **Normalize discussions of pain-related worry.**
  - You can use terms like "stress" as a stand-in for worry, fear, and anxiety until you have a better picture of the patient's symptoms. Most patients will understand the explanation of the pain–stress bidirectional cycle: *"As you know, pain is so complex and can affect your body*

and life in many different ways. We know that stress can affect pain intensity and vice versa—pain can cause stress in life."

- "Tell me about your stress levels lately."
- "Does your pain make you feel stressed?"
- "Do you ever notice that your stress makes your pain worse?"
- If you observe overt signs of anxiety—tight fists when they talk about work, jaw clenched as they discuss family, shoulders hunched to their ears—you can provide feedback on what you notice: "I notice that when you talked about the car accident, your voice changed and you started wringing your hands together like this." "Did you notice that your shoulders go up when you talk about whether you should go through with this next surgery?"
- **Provide education about the body and offer advice about fear-avoidance beliefs to correct misinformation.**
  - "You mentioned that you worry that an exercise program will make your degenerative disc disease worse. We know that spine degeneration is a normal part of aging. DDD is not terminal. Progression is determined by a number of factors, but also just genetics. Bed rest and avoiding activity does not prevent future degeneration. It's safe to load the spine with careful lifting and engage in your fun hobbies like camping—although that may occasionally cause some temporarily increased pain, it's not causing lasting damage."
  - "Back pain can have layers—it's not just the discs and nerves, but also inflammation and tightness in the paraspinal muscles, all under the magnifying glass of how we think about pain and if our nervous system is sensitive. Stretching and physical activity can actually help the pain by calming the nervous system—it's like you're teaching your body that movement is safe and it doesn't have to be on high alert all the time. You can start slowly and test the waters. What do you think about seeing a physical therapist who can guide you safely through the movements, little by little, to increase your confidence in your body again?"
- **Don't leap to the medication management route immediately due to polypharmacy risks.**
  - "You mentioned that you're waking up with pain and anxiety in the middle of the night and having trouble getting back to sleep. I certainly understand the desire for a medication to help you get that rest you're lacking."

- *"However, given your current opioid regimen, I'd like us to be cautious about adding in something else that's sedating. We also know that many sleep medications, even though they may help with quantity of sleep, don't always get people the quality of REM and deep sleep they need to really feel rested."*
- *"What if we put a pin in the prescription for now—we can revisit it later—and for one or two months really work on sleep hygiene and relaxation instead?"*
- **Discuss the relaxation response. Relaxation tools can trigger a physiologic cascade that actually counteracts the pain response.**
  - Mindfulness techniques like breath awareness, loving-kindness meditations, and body scans take daily practice to retrain the mind and body away from pain. Guided visualizations that incorporate the senses are often 10- to 20-minute exercises. Biofeedback-assisted relaxation takes training and equipment to measure heart rate, electroencephalography (EEG), skin conductance, or electromyography (EMG) readings. However, there are some quick tools you can demonstrate in office to help the anxious patient:
    - **Box breathing**, also known as four-square breathing (Figure 8.2)—Exhale to a count of four, hold your lungs empty for a four-count, inhale to four, and hold air in your lungs to a count of four before beginning the pattern again. You can do this for three to five breaths as a quick reset.

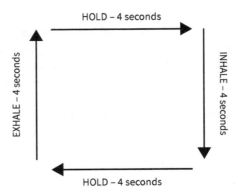

Figure 8.2 Box breathing

- **"Drop Three"**—This is a quick body scan from head to toe, with passive muscle relaxation ("dropping" or loosening) of (1) the jaw, (2) the shoulders, and (3) the hands (unclench fists and turn hands palm up).
- 5-4-3-2-1 **"grounding technique"**—Born out of trauma counseling and often used in patients with PTSD, grounding techniques help to refocus a patient on the present moment. This technique is about noticing small details of one's surroundings using each of the senses:
  - What are five things you can see?
  - What are four things you can feel?
  - What are three things you can hear?
  - What are two things you can smell?
  - What is one thing you can taste?

References

1. Ma Q, Qui W, Fu H, Sun X. Uncertain is worse: modulation of anxiety on pain anticipation by intensity uncertainty: evidence from the ERP study. *Neuroreport* 2018;29(12):1023–1029.
2. Grupe DW, Nitschke JB. Uncertainty and anticipation in anxiety: an integrated neurobiological and psychological perspective. *Nat Rev Neurosci* 2013;14(7):488–501.
3. Anxiety and Depression Association of America. Facts & Statistics. 2018. https://adaa.org/about-adaa/press-room/facts-statistics
4. American Psychiatric Association. *Diagnostic and Statistical Manual of Mental Disorders*. 5th ed. Arlington, VA: American Psychiatric Association, 2013.
5. Hauser W, Wolfe F. The somatic symptom disorder in DSM 5 risks mislabelling people with major medical diseases as mentally ill. *J Psychosom Res* 2013;75(6):586–587.
6. Toussaint A, Murray AM, Voight K, Herzog A, Gierk B, Kroenke K, Rief W, Henningsen P, Löwe B. Development and validation of the Somatic Symptom Disorder-B Criteria Scale (SSD-12). *Psychosom Med* 2015;78(1):5–12.
7. Munn Z, Moola S, Lisy K, Riitano D, Murphy F. Claustrophobia in magnetic resonance imaging: a systematic review and meta-analysis. *Radiography* 2015;21(2):e59–e63.

8. Edmonds JC, Yang H, King TS, Sawyer DA, Rizzo A, Sawyer AM. Claustrophobic tendencies and continuous positive airway pressure therapy non-adherence in adults with obstructive sleep apnea. *Heart Lung* 2015;44(2):100–106.

9. Vlaeyen JW, Kole-Snijders AM, Boeren RG, van Eck H. Fear of movement/(re) injury in chronic low back pain and its relation to behavioral performance. *Pain* 1995;62:363–372.

10. Vlaeyen JW, Kole-Snijders AM, Rotteveel AM, Ruesink R, Heuts PH. The role of fear of movement/(re)injury in pain disability. *J Occup Rehabil* 1995;5(4):235–252.

11. Vlaeyen JW, Linton SJ. Pain-related fear and its consequences in chronic musculoskeletal pain. Fear avoidance and its consequences in chronic musculoskeletal pain: a state of the art. *Pain* 2000;85:317–332.

12. Clark LA, Watson D, Mineka S. Temperament, personality, and the mood and anxiety disorders. *J Abnorm Psychol* 1994;103(1):103–116.

13. Eccleston C, Crombez, G. Pain demands attention: a cognitive-affective model of the interruptive function of pain. *Psychol Bull* 1999;125:356–366.

14. Crombez G, Vlaeyen JW, Heuts PH, Lysens R. Pain-related fear is more disabling than pain itself: evidence on the role of pain-related fear in chronic back pain disability. *Pain* 1999;80:329–339.

15. Zale EL, Lange KL, Fields SA, Ditre JW. The relation between pain-related fear and disability: a meta-analysis. *J Pain* 2013;14:1019–1030.

16. Vlaeyen JW, Linton SJ. Fear-avoidance model of chronic musculoskeletal pain: 12 years on. *Pain* 2012;153:1144–1147.

17. Crombez G, Eccleston C, Van Damme S, Vlaeyen JWS, Karoly P. Fear-avoidance model of chronic pain: the next generation. *Clin J Pain* 2012;28(6):475–483.

18. Ochsner KN, Ludlow DH, Knierim K, Hanelin J, Ramachandran T, Glover GC, Mackey SC. Neural correlates of individual differences in pain-related fear and anxiety. *Pain* 2006;120:69–77.

19. Lundberg M, Grimby-Ekman A, Verbunt J, Simmonds MJ. Pain-related fear: a critical review of the related measures. *Pain Res Treat* 2011;2011:494196. doi:10.1155/2011/494196

20. Kori SH, Miller RP, Todd DD. Kinesiophobia: a new view of chronic pain behavior. *Pain Manage* 1990;3:35–43.

21. McCracken LM, Zayfert C, Gross RT. The Pain Anxiety Symptoms Scale: development and validation of a scale to measure fear of pain. *Pain* 1992;50(1):67–73.

22. Waddell G, Newton M, Henderson I, Somerville D, Main CJ, A Fear-Avoidance Beliefs Questionnaire (FABQ) and the role of fear-avoidance beliefs in chronic low back pain and disability. *Pain* 1993;52:157–168.

23. Neblett R, Mayer TG, Hartzell MM, Williams MJ, Gatchel RJ. The Fear-Avoidance Components Scale (FACS): development and psychometric evaluation of a new measure of pain-related fear avoidance. *Pain Pract* 2016;16(4):435–450.

24. Rainville J, Smeets R, Bendix T, Tveito TH, Poiraudeau S, Indahl AJ. Fear-avoidance beliefs and pain avoidance in low back pain—translating research into clinical practice. *Spine J* 2011;11(9):895–903.

25. Linton SJ, Vlaeyen J, Osteol R. The back pain beliefs of health care providers: are we fear avoidant? *J Occup Rehabil* 2002;12:223–232.

26. Rainville J, Carlson N, Polatin P, Gatchel RJ, Indahl A. Exploration of physicians' recommendations for activities in chronic low back pain. *Spine* 2000;25(17):2210–2220.

27. Borkovec TD, Robinson E, Pruzinsky T, Dupree JA. Preliminary exploration of worry: some characteristics and processes. *Behav Res Ther* 1983;21:9–16.

28. Davey GCL, Tallis F, eds. *Worrying: Perspectives on Theory, Assessment, and Treatment.* Chichester, UK: John Wiley and Sons Ltd., 1994.

29. Eccleston C, Crombez G. Worry and chronic pain: a misdirected problem solving model. *Pain* 2007;132:233-236.

30. Selye H. A syndrome produced by diverse nocuous agents. *Nature* 1936;138:32.

31. Hannibal KE, Bishop MD. Chronic stress, cortisol dysfunction, and pain: a psychoneuroendocrine rationale for stress management in pain rehabilitation. *Phys Ther* 2014;94(12):1816–1825.

32. Sousa N. The dynamics of the stress neuromatrix. *Mol Psychiatry* 2016;21(3):302–312.

33. Marin EI, Ressler KJ, Binder E, Nemeroff CB. The neurobiology of anxiety disorders: brain imaging, genetics, and psychoneuroendocrinology. *Psychiatr Clin North Am* 2009;32(3):549–575.

34. Kroenke K, Outcalt S, Krebs E, Bair MJ, Wu MS, Chumbler N, Yu Z. Association between anxiety, health-related quality of life and functional impairment in primary care patients with chronic pain. *Gen Hos Psychiatry* 2013;35(4):359–365.

35. Manchikanti L, Pampati V, Beyer C, Damron K, Barnhill RC. Evaluation of psychological status in chronic low back pain: comparison with general population. *Pain Physician* 2002;5(2):149–166.

36. Manchikanti L, Fellows B, Pampati V Beyer C, Damron K, Barnhill RC. Comparison of psychological status of chronic pain patient and the general population. *Pain Physician* 2002; 5:40–48.

37. Demyttenaere K, Bruffaerts R, Lee S, Posada-Villa J, Kovess V, Angermeyer MC, Levinson D, de Girolamo G, Nakane H, Mneimneh Z, Lara C, de Graaf R, Scott KM, Gureje O, Stein DJ, Haro JM, Bromet EJ, Kessler RC, Alonso J, von Korff M.

Mental disorders among persons with chronic back or neck pain: results from the World Mental Health Surveys. *Pain* 2007;129(3):332–342.

38. Asmundson GJG, Norto G, Allerdings M, Norton P, Larsen D. Post-traumatic stress disorder and work-related injury. *J Anxiety Disord* 1998;12:57–69.

39. Hickling EJ, Blanchard EB. Post-traumatic stress disorder and motor vehicle accidents. *J Anxiety Disord* 1992;6:285–291.

40. Perry S, Cella D, Falkenberg J, Heidrich G, Goodwin C. Pain perception in burn patients with stress disorders. *J Pain Symptom Manage* 1987;2:29–33.

41. Von Korff M, Crane P, Lane M, Miglioretti DL, Simon G, Saunders K, Stang P, Brandenburg N, Kessler R. Chronic spinal pain and physical-mental comorbidity in the United States: results from the National Comorbidity Survey Replication. *Pain* 2005;113(3):331–339.

42. Patel SK, Gozal YM, Saleh MS, Gibson JL, Karsy M, Mandybur GT. Spinal cord stimulation failure: evaluation of factors underlying hardware explantation. *J Neurosurg Spine* 2019 (Oct 4):1–6 [E-pub before print].

43. Schumann M, Townsend C. Chronic pain and anxiety: a treatment outcome comparison of patients with anxiety in an interdisciplinary pain rehabilitation program. *J Pain* 2013;14(4):S94.

44. Bair MJ, Wu J, Damush TM, Sutherland JM, Kroenke K. Association of depression and anxiety alone and in combination with chronic musculoskeletal pain in primary care patients. *Psychosom Med* 2008;70(8):890–897.

45. McLaughlin TP, Khandker RK, Kruzikas DT, Tummala R. Overlap of anxiety and depression in a managed care population: prevalence and association with resource utilization. *J Clin Psychiatry* 2006;67:1187–1193.

46. Lerman SF, Rudich Z, Brill S, Shalev H, Shahar G. Longitudinal associations between depression, anxiety, pain, and pain-related disability in chronic pain patients. *Psychosom Med* 2015;77(3):333–341.

47. Asmundson GJ, Katz J. Understanding the co-occurrence of anxiety disorders and chronic pain: state-of-the-art. *Depress Anxiety* 2009;26(10):888–901.

48. Simons LE, Moulton EA, Linnman C, Carpino E, Becerra L, Borsook D. The human amygdala and pain: evidence from neuroimaging. *Hum Brain Mapp* 2014;35(2):527–538.

49. Huang B, Dawson DA, Stinson FS, Hasin DS, Ruan W, Saha TD, et al. Prevalence, correlates, and comorbidity of nonmedical prescription drug use and drug use disorders in the United States: Results of the National Epidemiologic Survey on Alcohol and Related Conditions. *J Clin Psychiatry,* 2006;67(7):1062–1073.

50. Fenton MC, Keyes K, Geier T, Greenstein E, Skodol A, Krueger B, Grant BF, Hasin DS. Psychiatric comorbidity and the persistence of drug use disorders in the United States. *Addiction* 2012;107:599–609.

51. Grant BF, Stinson FS, Dawson DA, Chou SP, Dufour MC, Compton W, Pickering RP, Kaplan K. Prevalence and co-occurrence of substance use disorders and independent mood and anxiety disorders: results from the National Epidemiologic Survey on Alcohol and Related Conditions. *Arch Gen Psychiatry* 2004;61(8):807–816.

52. Becker WC, Sullivan LE, Tetrault JM, Desai RA, Fiellin DA. Non-medical use, abuse and dependence on prescription opioids among US adults: psychiatric, medical and substance use correlates. *Drug Alcohol Depend* 2008:94:38–47.

53. Fischer B, Lusted A, Roerecke M, Taylor B, Rehm J. The prevalence of mental health and pain symptoms in general population samples reporting nonmedical use of prescription opioids: a systematic review and meta-analysis. *J Pain* 2012;13:1029–1044.

54. Wasan AD, Butler SF, Budman SH, Benoit C, Fernandez K, Jamison RN. Psychiatric history and psychologic adjustment as risk factors for aberrant drug related behavior among patients with chronic pain. *Clin J Pain* 2007;23:307–315.

55. Feingold D, Brill S, Goor-Areyh I, Delayahu Y, Lev-Ran S. Misuse of prescription opioids among chronic pain patients suffering from anxiety: a cross-sectional analysis. *Gen Hosp Psychiatry* 2017;47:36–42.

56. Martins SS, Fenton MC, Keyes KM, Blanco C, Zhu H, Storr CL. Mood and anxiety disorders and their association with non-medical prescription opioid use and prescription opioid-use disorder: longitudinal evidence form the National Epidemiologic Study on Alcohol and Related Conditions. *Psychol Med* 2012;42(6):1261–1272.

57. Schepis TS, Hakes JK. Non-medical prescription use increases the risk for the onset and recurrence of psychopathology: results from the National Epidemiological Survey on Alcohol and Related Conditions. *Addiction* 2011;106(12):2146–2155.

58. Gressler LE, Martin BC, Hudson TJ, Painter JT. Relationship between concomitant benzodiazepine-opioid use and adverse outcomes among US veterans. *Pain* 2018;159(3):451–459.

59. Macleod J, Steer C, Tilling K, Cornish R, Marsden J, Millar T, Strang J, Hickman J. Prescription of benzodiazepines, z-drugs, and gabapentinoids and mortality risk in people receiving opioid agonist treatment: observational study based on the UK Clinical Practice Research Datalink and Office for National Statistics death records. *PLoS Med* 2019;16(11):e1002965. doi:10.1371/journal.pmed.1002965

60. Jann M, Kennedy WK, Lopez G. Benzodiazepines: a major component in unintentional prescription drug overdoses with opioid analgesics. *J Pharm Pract* 2014;27(1):5–16.

61. Dasgupta N, Funk MJ, Proescholdbell S, Hirsch A, Ribisl KM, Marshall S. Cohort study of the impact of high-dose opioid analgesics on overdose mortality. *Pain Med* 2016;17(1):85–98.

62. Dowell D, Haegerich TM, Chou R. CDC guideline for prescribing opioids for chronic pain—United States, 2016. *JAMA* 2016;315(15):1624–1645.

63. George S, Wittmer VT, Rillingim RB, Robinson ME. Comparison of graded exercise and graded exposure clinical outcomes for patients with chronic low back pain. *J Orthop Sports Phys Ther* 2010;40(11):694–704.

64. Kabat-Zinn J, Hanh T. *Full Catastrophe Living: Using the Wisdom of Your Body and Mind to Face Stress, Pain, and Illness.* New York: Random House, 2009.

65. Davidson RJ, Kabat-Zinn J, Schumacher J, Rosenkranz M, Muller D, Santorelli SF, Urbanowski F, Harrington A, Bonus K, Sheridan JF. Alterations in brain and immune function produced by mindfulness meditation. *Psychosom Med* 2003;65(4):564–570.

66. Black DS, Slavich GM. Mindfulness meditation and the immune system: a systematic review of randomized controlled trials. *Ann N Y Acad Sci* 2016;(1):13–24.

67. Asmundson GJ, Fetzner MG, DeBoer LB, Powers MB, Otto MW, Smits J. Let's get physical: a contemporary review of the anxiolytic effects of exercise for anxiety and its disorders. *Depress Anxiety* 2013;30(4):362–373.

68. Spitzer RL, Kroenke K, Williams JB, Lowe B. A brief measure for assessing generalized anxiety disorder: the GAD-7. *Arch Intern Med* 2006;166:1092–1097.

Further Reading

McGeary D, McGeary C, Nabity P. Treating patients with somatic symptom and related disorders. In Turk DC, Gatchel RJ (eds.), *Psychological Approaches to Pain Management: A Practitioner's Handbook.* 3rd ed. New York: Guilford Press, 2018:499–514.

Salas E, Kishino N, Dersh J, Gatchel RJ. Psychological disorders and chronic pain: are there cause and effect relationships? In Turk DC, Gatchel RJ (eds.), *Psychological Approaches to Pain Management: A Practitioner's Handbook.* 3rd ed. New York: Guilford Press, 2018:25–50.

Turk DC. A cognitive-behavioral perspective on the treatment of individuals experiencing chronic pain. In Turk DC, Gatchel RJ (eds.), *Psychological Approaches to*

Pain Management: A Practitioner's Handbook. 3rd ed. New York: Guilford Press, 2018:115–137.

Vlaeyen JWS, den Hollander M, de Jong J, Simons L. Exposure in vivo for pain-related fear. In Turk DC, Gatchel RJ (eds.), *Psychological Approaches to Pain Management: A Practitioner's Handbook.* 3rd ed. New York: Guilford Press, 2018:177–204.

Wolf LD, Otis JD. Treating patients with posttraumatic stress disorder and chronic pain. In Turk DC, Gatchel RJ (eds.), *Psychological Approaches to Pain Management: A Practitioner's Handbook.* 3rd ed. New York: Guilford Press, 2018:515–529.

Relaxation and Mindfulness Meditation Resources

Davis M, Eshelman ER, McKay M. *The Relaxation and Stress Reduction Workbook.* Oakland, CA: New Harbinger Publications, 2008.

Kabat-Zinn J, Hanh T. *Full Catastrophe Living: Using the Wisdom of Your Body and Mind to Face Stress, Pain, and Illness.* New York: Random House, 2009.

Siegel RD. *The Mindfulness Solution: Everyday Practices for Everyday Problems.* New York: Guilford Press, 2010.

Free online Mindfulness-Based Stress Reduction (MBSR) course: www.palousemindfulness.com

Free Breath Pacer Apps

- Breathe2Relax app from the National Center for Telehealth & Technology
- Kardia—Deep Breathing Relaxation

Free Guided Meditations

- https://counselingcenter.utah.edu/services/audiomindfulness.php   (Body Awareness, Calm Place, Deep Breathing, Mindful Breathing)
- https://www.uclahealth.org/marc/body.cfm?id=22

Free Basic/Paid Membership Mindfulness Apps (for Android and Apple)

- InsightTimer
- Calm
- Headspace

Tai Chi for Arthritis with Dr. Paul Lam: https://taichiforhealthinstitute.org/programs/tai-chi-for-arthritis/

9
The Angry Patient

Daniel M. Doleys

Case: The Angry Patient

Let's consider "Herman," a 55-year-old male with longstanding chronic low back pain. He's been under your care for a year, although he has seen several other physicians before you. Although he is generally compliant with your treatment plan, he never seems satisfied and always appears irritable and unhappy. Your front-office staff and medical assistants dread interacting with his scowl and gruff demeanor. Your treatment recommendations are often countered with something to the effect of "I've already tried that and IT DIDN'T WORK!" His pain complaints have been somewhat nonspecific and the pain-related pathology is not overly impressive. He insists that the medications you have prescribed are not adequately addressing his pain and his quality of life is reduced. Although he is on a moderate opioid dose, he demands that you increase it. When his request is declined, he angrily accuses you of not caring, not wanting to help, or not believing him, and says you are "just like every other doctor" he's seen. He's accused you of being in practice only for the money. He demands that you "must do something!"

Challenge: Developing Self-Awareness and Avoiding Fighting Fire with Fire

If you have not had a "Herman" in your practice, you simply have not been in practice long enough. At times the angry patient can remind one of the line from Shakespeare's *Macbeth*: "Life is a tale told by an idiot, full of sound and fury, signifying nothing" (Act 5, Scene 5). Yet, at the same time, there is something unnerving about such a patient. You may feel sad, guilty, fearful, and resentful all at the same time. It can feel as though the patient is trying to manipulate you by provoking an inappropriate response, and in some cases this may be true. The urge to discharge such a patient is all but unavoidable. However, we may have experienced or heard of colleagues' patients exacting revenge by blogging, posting one-sided reviews on the internet, or filing complaints with the medical board. Vague and ambiguous diagnoses, unmet expectations for treatment, conflict with insurance companies or employers, forced medication changes, loss of income, and history of head trauma are potential contributing factors.

Anger also plays a role in a patient's decision to bring legal action. The likelihood of patients initiating legal action is increased if they feel coerced, if they experienced anger from and/or for the clinician, and if they felt the physician was motivated primarily by financial reasons.[1] Conversely, the likelihood of a patient initiating legal action is 78% less for those indicating that they "trusted" their doctor.[1]

Primary care clinicians are also at risk for experiencing violence from some patients. According to Cosio,[2] nearly 75% of workplace assaults take place in the health care setting.[3] Sixty-three percent of physicians reported that they had experienced abuse or violence during the previous year and 11% reported experiencing some form of verbal abuse in their practice on a daily basis.[4] The risk of abusive or violent interactions appears to be increased if the clinician confronts a patient over drug-seeking behavior or drug use or does not validate a patient's disability status.[4-6] If a patient has a history of violence, poor impulse control, and/or a history of opioid use disorder, the risk is likely increased.[2] These statistics are not meant to discourage or frighten the provider; rather, they are presented merely to highlight the need for strategies to manage the angry patient and volatile situations to mitigate escalation.

The clinician's understanding and view of chronic pain can influence their interpretation of, and response to, the patient's behavior. Consider the patient who presents with a flat affect yet reports pain that is disproportionate to the physical findings. He is complaining of poor sleep and inactivity. Watching television or surfing the internet consumes his waking hours. He is apprehensive about returning to work for fear of re-injury and worsening pain. He expounds on the severity of his pain as well as his depressed mood and anxiousness. What is your initial impression? It is most likely one of several, including that (a) he is drug-seeking, (b) he is malingering, (c) he is exhibiting hysterical responding, or (d) he is a suffering patient with the inability to successfully cope. As discussed in Chapter 2, our automatic schemas and unconscious interpretations influence our initial impression. The susceptibility to these implicit influences on our responses to the angry and difficult patient is certainly no different, if not more salient. Consider the following two scenarios that are not uncommonly heard in the pain management practice:

> *Doc, I know they said there was nothing new on the MRI and another surgery is not recommended. You aren't listening to me! You aren't doing anything to help me. I hurt like hell. I can't fish and hunt. It takes hours or days to cut the grass and I am always snapping at my wife. You need to do something! I really don't give a damn about those guidelines and I am tired of hearing about them. Why are you making me suffer because of a few bad apples?*
> or . . .
> *Doc, I know they said the cancer is gone, but I swear, it feels like it is still there. The chemo and radiation therapy were terrible, let alone going through the surgery. The pain is a constant reminder. I still find myself avoiding an activity that aggravates it. It sure would help if I could have some extra pain medicine so I can at least get some enjoyment out life.*

In order to respond effectively to emotionally charged interactions, clinicians must be aware of their own predispositions and predilections. After all, the patient–clinician relationship is dynamic, and anger can readily trigger defensiveness from the clinician, which in turn can be projected back as anger to the patient. This is a very automatic and human response. To see ways in which the expressed anger from others can trigger our own emotions, let's take a look at examples we might have experienced personally. Has your spouse or loved one ever come to you with "*You never* take the trash out!" or "*You always* get on the phone just when I need to talk to you. *You* don't care about what I need to say."

What do you notice? We don't often think about it, but a heated statement coming from another person that begins with "you" and continues with extremes such as "always" or "never" is like verbal finger-pointing. It can immediately elicit feelings of defensiveness, which is only exacerbated when such statements are coupled with blanket appraisals that we know to be untrue (e.g., "you don't care"). As a result, we may respond angrily to "nip" such a false accusation "in the bud." Unfortunately, this likely only foments the other party's anger and escalates the overall conflict.

Clinician Context: Maintaining Awareness of One's Own Emotions as a First Step Toward Productive Resolution

As discussed previously in this book, developing self-awareness and mindfulness of your own emotions in a given context can facilitate effective communication and cultivation of empathy, even in the most interpersonally challenging situations. Emotional predispositions, especially empathy, are known to change with time and experience and in ways of which we are not fully aware. Empathy, for example, has been described to have several types, including cognitive, emotional, trait, and state empathy.[7] Neuroimaging studies have uncovered different brain activation patterns when the subject explicitly attends to and evaluates the feelings of others.[8] However, studies that have followed physicians over time reveal a decline in empathy, which can begin during medical training and before independent practice.[7,9,10] The burden of patient care, the business demands of a successful practice, changing regulations, and lack of balance in personal versus professional life can certainly increase the difficulty of maintaining focus on empathetic communication. Being aware of what type of patient "pushes your buttons" and self-monitoring your response can save time, conserve your emotional resources, maintain the therapeutic alliance, and move the patient toward progress.

Being a clinician, especially a physician, demands a high degree of judgment, often in situations where time is in short supply and deliberate, reflective thought is an impractical luxury. Coupled with a reduced level of empathy,[9] physicians may find themselves with lower positive and adaptive attitudes and increased cynicism toward patients. This can lead providers to respond to distressed and angry patients in kind—that is, with anger and distress as well. On the other hand, physicians who can regulate their emotions can mitigate the intensifying emotions that may develop in a patient–provider dynamic. Moreover, evidence also suggests that emotional regulation may aid in better assessment of pain in others. Exposure to the suffering and pain of others naturally increases our own stress response; however, physicians who can effectively regulate their own emotions appear to experience a reduced stress response in such contexts.[11] In turn, lower negative emotional arousal allows physicians to be more empathetic, with greater ability to focus on effective problem-solving strategies for the perceived barrier at hand.

How patients express anger can range widely, and learning the various signs of anger can help you use them as cues to switch into a more mindful and self-aware mode of interacting. Anger exists on a continuum, extending from mild frustration to hostility or even rage. Some patients will internalize their anger, and this can lead to the development or worsening of clinical symptoms. Often these patients may make more indirect or passive expressions of their anger (e.g., *"Whatever; you're the doctor"*) or engage in a behavior that is sabotaging, such as purposeful noncompliance. Other patients may readily express their anger, verbally "unloading" in the exam room. Patients may become angry about interactions with office staff, billing issues, or your proposed treatment plan, with the latter especially common in the context of opioid therapy. Anger may be the only emotion, or it may occur as part of a bigger problem such as mild traumatic brain injury, dementia, depression, or a personality disorder. Some patients use their anger to provoke an uncharacteristic and perhaps unprofessional response from the clinician, which the patient finds reinforcing as a means of exerting control in a seemingly uncontrollable situation, such as their chronic pain.

Before going further, an important point to make is that anger itself is not necessarily bad, wrong, or an emotion that should be forbidden. Anger is a very normal part of our emotional repertoire. Like pain, it can serve as an important signal that something is wrong. Anger can direct our attention toward true injustices, motivate us to find a solution to a problem, or overcome a barrier to a goal. However, when uncontrolled, it can impede social, occupational, and psychological functioning and well-being. There are several signs of uncontrolled anger: having a "short fuse" or easily losing one's temper, being impatient and restless, becoming easily annoyed or agitated, having verbal outbursts, having trouble concentrating, and obsessing about an event, person, or situation. At times, these behaviors can become quite egregious and disruptive.

The first priority is the safety of your staff and patients, followed by preserving the therapeutic relationship with the angry patient to allow for productive resolutions. When clinicians encounter a disruptive and hostile patient, Box 9.1 lists some initial steps that can deescalate the situation.

Box 9.1 Initial steps when encountering patient hostility

- Do not provoke or argue with the patient.
- If needed, excuse yourself for a moment to collect your thoughts.
- Scoot back. Uncross your arms. Create some physical space between you and the patient. Never stand over the patient.
- Remain calm and supportive.
- Do not patronize or belittle the patient.
- Above all, do not touch the patient.
- If the patient remains disruptive or refuses to leave when asked, call 911.

Patient Context: Factors Contributing to Anger and How Anger Impacts Pain

Anger is certainly not rare among individuals with chronic pain who are seeking care. The rate at which patients express dissatisfaction with their pain management ranges from 15% to as much as 42%.[12] Approximately 70% of patients with chronic pain report feelings of anger, with 62% reporting anger toward health care providers, 39% toward significant others, and 30% toward insurance companies.[13] There are many reasons patients become angry and frustrated, including feeling abandoned and unfairly treated by the medical community, having expectations of a "cure" unmet, and fear of pain from therapeutic increases in activity. Perceived unnecessarily long wait times, a provider's refusal to order "feel-good" therapies such as massage or equipment (e.g., specialty mattresses), forced opioid reduction, and inappropriate reactions on the part of office staff may also ignite and inflame the already existing anger. Patients who are involved with open legal matters related to an injury (e.g., worker's compensation) may view the accident that caused their injury as a result of inappropriate safety measures. Their anger may be associated with sense of entitlement to reparation (financially or emotionally), couched in a desire for retribution that may be displaced onto the clinician.

Anger can broadly be perceived as the emotional response to some perceived barrier that interferes with reaching a reward. This perceived reward could be relief of pain and pursuit of important life activities. When efforts toward goals are frustrated, we may respond with anger in different ways, depending on our personality as well as the beliefs and attitudes we hold about the world. This will be much of the focus of this chapter, yet the clinician must also consider anger in the context of aberrant drug behaviors. For instance, a patient who is diverting a prescription for financial gain will likely become angry when that goal is frustrated by a reduction in the dose or change to a drug with a lower street value. This should be teased apart from the compliant "legitimate" patient whose anger may be in response to a sudden, unforeseen, and unjustified change in treatment such as necessary medication tapers to reduce medical risk.

Pain Factors

In some instances, anger has been closely associated with specific types of pain. About 10% of patients with arthritis, back/neck pain, headaches, and other chronic pain conditions expressed anger and met criteria for intermittent explosive disorder.[14,15] Patients with migraines or tension headaches tend have higher anger levels and poorer anger control.[16] Others[12] have reported anger in 27% of patients with diabetic neuropathy compared to 42% in those with peripheral neuropathy. Patients scoring higher on measures of hostility tend to complain of chest pain,[17] and anger appears to be a predictor of pain in those with spinal cord injuries.[18] Anger also correlates with greater pain intensity and pain duration in patients with cancer-related pain.[19,20]

Anger has also been associated with greater muscle tension, pain severity, and pain behaviors in patients with chronic pain.[21] Indeed, uncontrolled anger has even been associated with higher levels of inflammatory markers such as C-reactive protein (CRP) and interleukin-6 (IL-6),[22] and IL-6 can induce muscle and joint hyperalgesia as well as injury-induced hyperalgesia.[23–25] Therefore, anger may be a predisposing, precipitating, exacerbating, or perpetuating factor in pain.

The severity of the injury may also be a factor contributing to anger. Losing the distal end of the fifth finger or suffering a one-level surgically corrected disc herniation is far different from experiencing paralysis, brain trauma, amputation, or other injury with life-altering implications. Individuals whose livelihoods were previously in manual labor or blue-collar jobs tend to be more vulnerable to grief and anger. Their transferable skills are likely to be minimal and a perceived inability to pursue previously reinforcing and "identity-relevant" activities leads them to be become compromised both emotionally and psychologically. As a result, an individual may experience a two-part grief response. On one hand, the patient grieves the loss of a "life that was"—a rewarding and functionally active life. On the other, the patient may ruminate on the "life that was to be," grieving for the loss of future plans, goals, and expectations.

Personality Factors

One of the most recognized theories of anger is the state-trait personality theory of anger.[26,27] *State* anger refers to transient subjective feelings of anger and accompanying physiologic arousal occurring in response to a specific and present situation. State anger can fluctuate and vary in intensity over a relatively short period of time. On the other hand, *trait* anger is considered to be a unique personality disposition toward anger proneness. Individuals with trait anger tend to become more easily angered, respond with more intense anger when provoked, and express anger in a less adaptive and functional manner.[26,27]

One's ability to self-regulate the arousal accompanying anger is associated with mental and physical well-being.[28] Individuals may attempt to regulate the negative experience of anger by suppressing that emotion, termed "anger-in," or by direct verbal or physical expression, termed "anger-out."[29] The direct expression used by those with traits toward anger-out may include verbal insults/aggression, sarcasm, arguing, physical expressions (e.g., striking out, slamming doors), or what is commonly referred to "losing one's temper."

In the context of pain, trait anger-out is associated with increased sensitivity to both acute and chronic pain.[30] There is functional overlap in the cortical areas that process pain and anger, particularly in the areas that process emotion, such as the limbic regions.[31] Furthermore, the endogenous opioid system plays a role in regulating activity among these regions. Thus, a dysfunctional opioid system with reduced inhibitory activity may serve as the nexus between trait anger-out and pain.[31,32] Bolstering this connection is the observation that opioids are effective in controlling agitation[33,34] and impulsiveness.[35] Further, the reduction or discontinuation of opioids may be associated with what has been termed a "protracted abstinence syndrome" that can include agitation.[36]

Elevated trait anger-out in the absence of direct expression may exacerbate pain sensitivity,[30] and anger expression can activate the endogenous opioid system, resulting in diminished pain.[21] In contrast, when individuals with higher trait anger-out attempt to suppress their anger, they experience increased pain responsiveness.[37] Thus, for individuals with a predominately expressive anger regulation style, behavioral anger expression may be functional and reinforcing. Thus, it is helpful to consider that angry patients are engaging in behavior that has worked for them, perhaps by providing some relief, and it is therefore a cycle that is difficult to disentangle. The goal should not be to help them avoid or suppress their anger, but rather to find ways to express anger in more assertive, adaptive, and healthy ways. This can be accomplished in the psychotherapeutic strategies identified in Chapter 2 when the patient is referred to work with a pain psychologist or other available qualified mental health provider.

Perceived Injustice

Patients with chronic pain often become frustrated with their inability to participate in valued, self-enhancing, and goal-driven activities. Anger can emerge from the resulting reduction in quality of life and diminished self-esteem. Anger is often generated and made worse by externalizing blame. For the patient with chronic pain, the targets may include medical and mental health providers, the legal system, third-party payors, employers, significant others, God, or even the whole world.[13,38] Patients' anger may also arise from perceived injustice—appraising the losses accompanying their chronic pain as unfair and irreparable, and externalizing the blame for this misfortune.[39,40]

Perceived injustice is associated with poorer coping skills, more severe pain, maladaptive pain behaviors, greater depression, and poorer outcomes in acute and chronic pain populations.[39] A patient's sense of injustice is also related to broader, long-term measures, including long-term work absence and reduced likelihood of returning to work.[39] Perceived injustice was identified as a unique predictor of posttraumatic symptom chronicity among whiplash injury patients.[41] Patients who experience greater perceived injustice also tend to have more depression, greater pain interference, and reduced satisfaction with life.[42] Lastly, perceived injustice in the context of pain is associated with higher levels of pain catastrophizing and interference with adjusting to limitations in an adaptive fashion.[43]

One question that arises is whether the experience of chronic pain leads to perceived injustice, or whether some individuals have a more enduring tendency to interpret negative life events as unjust when they are encountered. There is some evidence for the latter, as otherwise pain-free individuals with trait-like perceived injustice rated experimental pain as more severe and reported greater sadness and anger related to the painful experience.[44] More specifically, anger explained the relationship between perceived injustice and pain severity, meaning that a perceived injustice was related to anger, which in turn predicted pain severity.[44] In this regard, patients with a propensity to interpret negative life events as unjust may be more likely to respond or cope with anger when those events arise. To the patient, acknowledging improvement in pain may be viewed as letting those responsible "off the hook." In this way, the patient may unconsciously interpret exhibiting greater pain severity and disability is a means of punishing the person they perceive as responsible for their injury.

Conversely, maintaining a sense of a just world, despite personal adversity, might protect against undue psychological distress when exposed to a situation involving pain. One's spiritual or religious predilection may play a role in formulating core justice beliefs, injustice appraisals, fairness, and forgiveness.[45] It seems noteworthy that an adaptive relationship between pain, perceived injustice, and a personal just-world belief can, in part, be accounted for by continuing to pursue valued and desired life activities despite pain.[45] This appears to reinforce the notion that, for all practical purposes, improved function and quality of life should take priority over changes in the numeric pain rating score as a treatment goal.

Communication: Strategies to Mitigate Anger and Maintain the Therapeutic Relationship

Table 9.1 offers suggested actions and responses when encountering the angry patient.

Encountering the angry patient can elicit a number of emotions within the provider, ranging from reflexive anger and frustration to even fear and intimidation. You can adopt a variety of strategies, both in your actions and verbal communication, that can deescalate the situation and resolve the situation. In some cases, this may be relatively simple. For example, a simple response like *"I am sorry the prescription was not correct. We can take care of that right now"* may be a sufficient way to handle the patient who angrily complains about what is a simple miscommunication issue. While other cases may prove more challenging, it is our experience that most situations can be handled with some "on-site" problem-solving.

Table 9.1 Suggested actions and responses when encountering the angry patient

Suggested Actions	Suggested Response
Avoid public interaction	Let's go into my office (examination room) and discuss the issue.
Have a witness	If you do not mind, I have asked my nurse to join us. Perhaps she can help with the problem.
Allow the patient's narrative	Why don't you go ahead and tell me about your concerns.
Do not dismiss the issue	Well, I can certainly see how your view of it could be upsetting.
Be supportive, but assertive	I understand the issues, but I think there are other ways of interpreting it and other ways of handling it.
Offer options	Let me outline a couple of options. Some may or may be not be acceptable, but I want you to be aware of them so we can have a reasonable discussion. I would be interested in what you think would resolve this.
Termination	It does not appear that we are going to be able to resolve this issue. If you wish, I would be glad to provide you the names of other clinicians (clinics) you may want to consider and can assist with transferring of your records. But I would greatly appreciate it if you would behave appropriately while in the office area.

When faced with an angry patient, there are several actions that can be beneficial (Table 9.2). Avoiding public interaction (e.g., in clinic hallways or waiting areas) yet having a member of your clinic team present during the interaction is good practice from recordkeeping, legal, and safety standpoints. Allowing patients to state their concern without dismissing the issue will send a message of empathy and will be sufficient to deescalate anger in many cases. Lastly, many patients who struggle with anger may feel a lack of control in the situation. Providing options from which they can choose to resolve the matter, as long as they are clinically appropriate to their treatment plan, can give them a sense of control and efficacy.

Unfortunately, some cases are not so easily managed. This is particularly the case when patients are not aware that their anger and the manner in which it is expressed is inappropriate or is a recurring problem that interferes with functioning. The suggestion that they would benefit from some counseling, particularly when inserted *during* an angry encounter, may simply inflame the situation. In subsequent encounters or when the patient is calm, noting the connection between stress, anger, and pain can open the door to referrals for psychotherapy to learn more helpful coping strategies. However, for the willing patient, a brief intervention from you can also be

Table 9.2 Approach to the treatment of anger

Objective	Treatment Strategy
Develop self-awareness	Use of psychotherapy, especially cognitive–behavioral therapy (CBT), to (a) recognize internal and external triggers, (b) identify how one behaves when angry, (c) recognize self-defeating negative thoughts that lie behind anger flares, (d) cope better with difficult life situations, and c) resolve conflicts
Modify the patient's response to anger	Patients can be taught how to use (a) relaxation techniques (e.g., diaphragmatic breathing, progressive muscle relaxation), (b) cognitive restructuring to alter maladaptive thoughts, and (c) problem-solving and distraction (e.g., exercising or engaging in a hobby).
Learn to differentiate passive, passive-aggressive, aggressive, and assertive communication styles.	Provide ways to (a) learn how to express angry feelings in an assertive manner, (b) make one's needs clear without hurting others, and (c) be assertive without being "pushy" or demanding.

Adapted from reference 2.

helpful. There are at least three approaches to treating anger in the chronic pain setting (see Table 9.2).

Patients with certain personality disorders, such as borderline personality disorder or other DSM "Cluster B" personality traits, are driven to create conflict and chaos. They may sabotage their own treatment as a means of engaging you in a debate—one you can never win. In these cases, setting appropriate emotional boundaries may feel like you are divesting professional responsibility, particularly in a helping profession, but in reality this will help the patient build a sense of ownership and self-efficacy over their pain management program. Outlining options, indicating what can and will be offered to the patient, and the willingness to refer them to another setting, may be appropriate in these situations.

The language used when interacting with the angry patient is also important. In the beginning of the this chapter, we highlighted how the emotional dynamic of a conflict can be intensified when verbalizing a complaint (or countering one coming from another person) with the use of "you" or sweeping statements such as "always" or "never." In general, the use of "I-statements" versus "you-statements" can help prevent an escalation in anger. The use of "I-statements" is an assertive communication strategy that can lower the defensiveness of the other party (therefore non-aggressive) while also allowing the communicator to state their own needs and concerns clearly (non-passive).

Let's compare the following two responses to a patient who states angrily that you are not helping and in fact are making her pain worse:

1. *"You need to calm down. You are overreacting. This is my practice and I will decide what is best. If you don't like it, you are free to leave."*
2. *"I see you are frustrated and I understand that you are not happy with your current treatment. However, under the circumstances, it is the best we can offer. If you feel the need to explore other options, I will be glad to assist in any way I can."*

With the first response, the patient may reflexively become more defensive and feel that her complaints are being devalued and dismissed. The use of an "I-statement" in the second response sends the message that you are only speaking from your point of view, without judgment to her concern. This also presents an opportunity to use empathetic listening, which can reveal other underlying reasons for a patient's anger. What may seem like a minor conflict or inconvenience for the patient from your perspective may be serving as an avenue through which a patient's larger stressors are becoming manifest. The patient's actions may reflect upheaval in other areas of her life, such as divorce or other relationship problems, financial stress, or other psychosocial stressors. A busy clinic will often not allow for the time to sort these issues out, though allowing patients to give their narrative for a few minutes can be effective. It can provide the basis for some clarification and an opportunity to offer assistance via a referral to a pain psychologist.

There will be occasions when patients are so disruptive to the office that discharge may be necessary. This is frequently met by various accusations of medical malpractice and the threat of legal action. In all cases, it is important to (a) document the interaction thoroughly in the medical record, (b) provide a discharge letter, (c) provide instruction for tapering of medications, (d) offer to transfer records with the appropriate request, (e) indicate where to seek alternative treatment (e.g., contacting the local medical society for other pain physicians), and (f) provide instructions as to seeking emergency care if needed. Verbally challenging or attempting to talk over such patients is likely to only escalate the conflict. Sometimes, the best way to win a tug-of-war is to let go of the rope.

To the extent possible, interactions with a volatile patient should be done away from other patients. The likelihood of an angry patient becoming violent is often foretold by increasing demands, raising one's voice, clenched fists, using abusive and profane language, restlessness, or slamming or attacking objects. Physical contact with the patient or engaging in a "shouting match" should be avoided at all costs. Having another staff member present during the interaction is advisable. In the presence of verbal or physical threats, the patient should be advised that unless they calm themselves, security or police will be called. The provider or clinic staff should follow through with calling authorities if necessary to ensure the safety of all parties. You should maintain a professional demeanor, but be prepared to take decisive action if called for.

Let's examine the role of an assertive I-statement in this context that also clearly states the ramifications of verbal or physical threats:

> *"I can appreciate your concerns, but raising your voice and yelling is not a way we can effectively resolve them. It is making the staff and other patients*

uncomfortable. I have done what I can to explain the situation. I must ask that you calm yourself or I will have to call the authorities."

Below are three situations that a provider might encounter when interacting with patients. The first sample case is about a patient injured on the job who required amputation. His views, and perhaps rightly so, are that the accident could have been avoided. The second sample case involves a patient who is not entirely compliant but feels entitled to medication changes. The third sample case involves a patient whose anger is likely associated with his pain-associated depression, poor coping, external locus of control, and feelings of helplessness.

Case 1

PATIENT: I told them repeatedly that someone was going to slip and fall on the gravel the way it was laid. I was ignored until I lost my leg. This did not have to happen! Somebody is going to pay!

CLINICIAN: I cannot imagine what that must to like. But you have to be careful not to get consumed by your anger.

PATIENT: You don't understand. I feel like a freak. Everyone stares at my prosthesis. The kids hesitate to come around me because they seem afraid of the stump. There is no way my wife can be attracted to me. It is probably only a matter of time before we divorce.

CLINICIAN: I think you are getting into too much "mind reading" and forecasting the future. If you dwell on this enough, you will come to believe it to be true and either start withdrawing or become very suspicious.

PATIENT: So you think I should just pretend it did not happen.

CLINICIAN: No, let me clarify what I mean. Unfortunately you cannot change the fact that it has happened, as unfair as it may be. However, you can decide how big of an impact it has on you now by how you deal with it. Also, there is evidence that your anger and stress can negatively affect your pain and how much benefit you experience from treatment.

This case is one experienced by the author (DMD). The patient's anger and need for "revenge" were palpable. Very little progress was made until the case was resolved legally. Every deposition and interview and ultimately the trial reinvigorated the patient's anger and sense of injustice. Individual therapy and consultation with his wife did provide some benefit for his functioning psychosocially, though the provider should not expect immediate change in the patient's coping and outlook. In general, our experience suggests that it may even take several years for patients to fully adjust to their "new normal."

Case 2

CLINICIAN: There have been concerns about your compliance with our medical agreement. I think we need to reevaluate your treatment and consider the options.

PATIENT: I suppose that means cutting my pain medicine. I don't know who you people think you are. I am barely getting by on what I have now. This whole opioid epidemic thing punishes people like me while the addicts and drug abusers run free. And by the way, I have done everything I am supposed to.

CLINICIAN: I hear your frustration, but you did fail to respond to our request to come in for a drug screen and pill count. That was our agreement.

PATIENT: I told you before—my voicemail was messed up. Do you expect me to sit by the phone all day just waiting for your call? I thought you wanted me to be busy. Oh, I forgot, you are the hotshot doctor and everyone is supposed to jump at your request.

CLINICIAN: There is also the matter of a drug screen that was positive for THC.

PATIENT: The stuff is legal in a lot of states. You complain about the opioid crisis and yet won't allow someone to use something that is safer and more effective. Besides, I told you before, it was probably from being around someone else that was using.

CLINICIAN: I understand you are angry . . .

PATIENT: No, you don't understand a damn thing! All you care about is following some stupid guideline. The fact that it destroys someone's life is of no concern. I suppose there is no sense in arguing because you have already made up your mind.

CLINICIAN: I want to outline what I think the options are for treatment. If they are not acceptable, I understand that you may want to relocate your care. If so, I will help in any way I can.

PATIENT: Oh, I get it now. All of this is just an effort to get rid of me. Well, good luck: it didn't work.

In Case 2, the patient is "looking for a fight." The situation was somewhat diffused by the clinician staying calm but at the same time being clear about the problems. Engaging in a verbal tug-of-war by arguing about the urine screen and his voicemail would be counterproductive and digress from the overall goal: getting the patient the most appropriate care to manage his pain. Moreover, proceeding in this way places the choice back with the patient. Rather than discharging the patient and risk being accused of abandoning the patient, one can present a very comprehensive treatment plan, which could include physical therapy, pain psychology, as well as medication adjustments. When this is done, one of two outcomes will occur: (1) the patient may agree, come into compliance, and make progress toward treatment goals or (2) the patient may reject the plan and essentially "discharge" themselves by not following up. Either way, the situation has been addressed professionally and appropriately without unnecessary confrontation or conflict.

Case 3

PATIENT: I just don't know what to do. Nothing is helping! My pain seems worse and I can't sleep. I don't want to be around anybody like this.
CLINICIAN: Have you had any episodes of being tearful?
PATIENT: Sure. Anyone living like this would.
CLINICIAN: Any thoughts of wanting to go to sleep and never wake up again, or of harming yourself?
PATIENT: I would be lying if I said the thought never crossed my mind.
CLINICIAN: Have you ever thought about how you would do it?
PATIENT: It has never gone that far, but there a lot of ways.
CLINICIAN: What has kept you from it?
PATIENT: I would never do that to my wife and kids. Besides, in my religion, suicide is considered to be unforgiveable. What's with all these questions? You think I'm crazy or something?
CLINICIAN: No, not at all. But there are a lot of signs of depression.
PATIENT: Of course I am depressed. Wouldn't you be in my situation? You get rid of this pain and everything will go back to normal.

CLINICIAN: I have no doubt that the pain is a big factor. In your situation, the depression is understandable and is getting to the point that it is making the pain and your ability to function more difficult.

PATIENT: So you think I need to see a shrink? That's all I need: another label and a bill!

CLINICIAN: Not exactly. But I do think we need to adjust your medicine. And, I want you to do me a favor and see Dr. Whyihurt. She is a specialist in pain and has helped several of my patients. Just see her once for a consultation. She can also guide me to know what I can do to help. Without some additional direction, we may both be spinning our wheels here.

In this relatively brief interaction, the clinician has performed a basic assessment for depression and suicidal risk. The patient is reassured that his situation is not uncommon and that he is not "crazy." By noting the doctor is not a "shrink" but a pain specialist and that seeing her would just be a consultation, some of the stigma and fear is removed. Indicating that this consult would also help you as the provider frames the request within a different perspective. The overall implications are that (a) pain and depression often coexist, (b) there are treatments that can help, and (c) the patient has to be willing to participate.

In conclusion, anger is a common patient response in the chronic pain setting, and the causes are many and varied. Perceived injustice, blame, or frustration over lack of goal achievement can constitute cognitive processes instrumental to the development and experience of anger. For some patients, the overt expression of anger may be reinforced by a reduction in pain intensity or perception, potentially developing into a pattern of behavior with biological underpinnings.[30,31] For others, anger is associated with the physical and emotional stresses of living with chronic pain, which may be displaced onto the clinician. Yet in other cases, anger may be the manifestation of a personality disorder or an attempt to manipulate the clinician in order to gain a sense of control.

Obtaining a psychological risk assessment early in the treatment trajectory can help to identify the emotional needs of patient, including anger. Preemptive measures such as frequency of visits, clarification of treatment goals, and implementing a treatment agreement can reduce ambiguity in expectations. Unacceptable behavior and its consequences, whether related to the use of prescribed medications or interpersonal conduct in the office, should be specified. In our setting, we conduct an orientation class for new patients that outlines clinic guidelines and expectations.

Adopting an appropriate style of interaction is crucial for the provider when caring for the angry patient. Becoming defensive, overly assertive, or confrontational is counterproductive and can damage the patient–provider relationship. The overarching goal in such situations is not "winning," but rather controlling and calming the situation with the primary focus on minimizing risk to office staff, other patients, and even the angry patient. There will be, of course, situations that cannot be satisfactorily resolved, and the clinical relationship will need to be dissolved. Even so, there is no reason this cannot be done in a professional and compassionate fashion.

References

1. Fishbain DA, Bruns D, Disorbio JM, Lewis JE. What are the variables that are associated with the patient's wish to sue his physician in patients with acute and chronic pain? *Pain Med* 2008;9:1130–1142.
2. Cosio D. Anger expression and chronic pain. *Pract Pain Manag* 2018;18(3). https://www.practicalpainmanagement.com/resources/clinical-practice-guidelines/anger-expression-chronic-pain
3. Phillips JP. Workplace violence against health care workers in the United States. *N Engl J Med* 2016;374:1661–1669.
4. Hobbs FD. Violence in general practice: a survey of general practitioners' views. *BMJ* 1991;302(6772):329–332.
5. Felton JS. Violence prevention at the health care site. *Occup Med* 1997;12(4):701–715.
6. Morrison JL, Lantos JD, Levinson W. Aggression and violence directed toward physicians. *J Gen Intern Med* 1998;13(8):556–561.
7. Newton BW. Walking a fine line: is it possible to remain an empathic physician and have a hardened heart? *Front Human Neurosci* 2013;7:233.
8. Fan Y, Duncan NW, de Greck M, Northoff G. Is there a core neural network in empathy? An fMRI based quantitative meta-analysis. *Neurosci Biobehav Rev* 2011;35(3):903–911.
9. Hojat M, Vergare M, Maxwell K, Brainard G, Herrine SK, Isenberg GA, Veloski J, Gonnella JS. The devil is in the third year: a longitudinal study of erosion of empathy in medical school. *Acad Med* 2009;84(9):1182–1191.
10. Neumann M, Edelhäuser F, Tauschel D, Fischer MR, Wirtz M, Woopen C, Haramati A, Scheffer C. Empathy decline and its reasons: a systematic review of studies with medical students and residents. *Acad Med* 2011;86(8):996–1009.

11. Decety J, Yang CY, Cheng Y. Physicians down-regulate their pain empathy response: an event-related brain potential study. *Neuroimage* 2008;50(4):1676–1682.

12. Parkoohi PI, Amirzadeh K, Mohabbati V, Abdollahifard G. Satisfaction with chronic pain treatment. *Anesth Pain Med* 2015;5(4):e23528.

13. Okifuji A, Turk DC, Curran SL. Anger in chronic pain: investigations of anger targets and intensity. *J Psychosom Res* 1999;47(1):1–12.

14. Fishbain DA, Goldberg M, Meagher BR, Steele R, Rosomoff H. Male and female chronic pain categorized by DSM-III psychiatric diagnostic criteria. *Pain* 1986;26(2):181–197.

15. McCloskey MS, Kleabir K, Berman ME, Chen EY, Coccaro EF. Unhealthy aggression: intermittent explosive disorder and adverse physical health outcomes. *Health Psychol* 2010;29(3):324–332.

16. Perozzo P, Savi L, Castelli L, Valfrè W, Lo Giudice R, Gentile S, Rainero I, Pinessi L. Anger and emotional distress in patients with migraine and tension-type headache. *J Headache Pain* 2005;6(5):392–399.

17. Tsouna-Hadjis E, Kallergis G, Agrios N, Zakopoulosa N, Lyropoulosa S, Liakosb A, Siderisc D, Stamatelopoulosa S. Pain intensity in non-diabetic patients with myocardial infarction or unstable angina. Its association with clinical and psychological features. *Int J Cardiol* 1998;67(2):165–169.

18. Summers JD, Rapoff MA, Varghese G, Porter K, Palmer RE. Psychosocial factors in chronic spinal cord injury pain. *Pain* 1991;47(2):183–189.

19. Glover J, Dibble SL, Dodd MJ, Miaskowski C. Mood states of oncology outpatients: does pain make a difference? *J Pain Symptom Manage* 1995;10(2):120–128.

20. Sela RA, Bruera E, Conner-Spady B, Cumming C, Walker C. Sensory and affective dimensions of advanced cancer pain. *Psychooncology* 2002;11(1):23–34.

21. Burns JW, Bruehl S, Chont M. Anger regulation style, anger arousal and acute pain sensitivity: Evidence for an endogenous opioid "triggering" model. *J Behav Med* 2014;37(4):642–653.

22. Coccaro EF, Lee R, Coussons-Read M. Elevated plasma inflammatory markers in individuals with intermittent explosive disorder and correlation with aggression in humans. *JAMA Psychiatry* 2014;71(2):158–165.

23. Atzeni F, Nucera V, Masala IF, Sarzi-Puttini P, Bonitta G. IL-6 involvement in pain, fatigue and mood disorders in rheumatoid arthritis and the effects of IL-6 inhibitor sarilumab. *Pharmacol Res* 2019;149:104402.

24. Manjavachi MN, Motta EM, Marotta DM, Leite DF, Calixto JB. Mechanisms involved in IL-6-induced muscular mechanical hyperalgesia in mice. *Pain* 2010;151(2):345–355.

25. Ding CP, Xue YS, Yu J, Guo YJ, Zeng XY, Wang JY. The red nucleus interleukin-6 participates in the maintenance of neuropathic pain induced by spared nerve injury. *Neurochem Res* 2016;41(11):3042–3051.

26. Spielberger CD, Jacobs G, Russell S, Crane R. Assessment of anger: the State-Trait Anger Scale. In Butcher JN, Spielberger CD (eds.), *Advances in Personality Assessment*. Vol. 2. Hillsdale, NJ: Erlbaum, 1983:159–187.

27. Spielberger CD, Johnson EH, Russell S, Crane RJ, Jacobs GA, Worden TJ. The experience and expression of anger: construction and validation of an anger expression scale. In Chesney MA, Rosenman RH (eds.), *Anger and Hostility in Cardiovascular and Behavioral Disorders*. New York: Hemisphere, 1985:5–30.

28. Gross JJ. The emerging field of emotion regulation: an integrative review. *Rev Gen Psychol* 1998;2:271–299.

29. Spielberger CD, Reheiser EC, Sydeman SJ. Measuring the experience, expression, and control of anger. In Kassinove H (ed.), *Anger Disorders: Definition, Diagnosis, and Treatment*. Washington, DC: Taylor & Francis, 1995:49–67.

30. Bruehl S, Burns JW, Chung OY, Chont M. Interacting effects of trait anger and acute anger arousal on pain: the role of endogenous opioids. *Psychosom Med* 2011;73(7):612–619.

31. Bruehl S, Burns JW, Chung OY, Chont M. Pain-related effects of trait anger expression: neural substrates and the role of endogenous opioid mechanisms. *Neurosci Biobehav Rev* 2009;33(3):475–491.

32. Bruehl S, Chung OY. Parental history of chronic pain may be associated with impairments in endogenous opioid analgesic systems. *Pain* 2006;124:287–294.

33. Husebo BS, Ballard C, Cohen-Mansfield J, Seifert R, Aarsland D. The response of agitated behavior to pain management in persons with dementia. *J Geriatr Psychiatry* 2014;22:708–717.

34. Brown R. Broadening the search for safe treatments in dementia agitation a possible role for low-dose opioids? *Int J Geriatr Psychiatry* 2010;25:1085–1086.

35. Love TM, Stohler CS, Zubieta JK. Positron emission tomography measures of endogenous opioid neurotransmission and impulsiveness traits in humans. *Arch Gen Psychiatry* 2009;66:1124–1134.

36. Manhapra A, Arias AJ, Ballantyne JC. The conundrum of opioid tapering in long-term opioid therapy for chronic pain: a commentary. *Subst Abus* 2018;39(2):152–161.

37. Burns JW, Quartana P, Bruehl S. Anger management style moderates effects of emotion suppression during initial stress on pain and cardiovascular responses during subsequent pain-induction. *Ann Behav Med* 2007;34:154–165.

38. Fernandez E, Wasan A. The anger of pain sufferers: attributions to agents and appraisals of wrongdoing. In Potegal M, Stemmler G, Spielberger C (eds.), *International Handbook of Anger: Constituent and Concomitant Biological, Psychological, and Social Processes*. New York: Springer, 2009:449–464.

39. Sullivan MJ, Adams H, Horan S, Maher D, Boland D, Gross R. The role of perceived injustice in the experience of chronic pain and disability: scale development and validation. *J Occup Rehabil* 2008;18:249–261.

40. Trost Z, Vangronsveld K, Linton S, Quartana J, Phillip J, Sullivan ML. Cognitive dimensions of anger in chronic pain. *Pain* 2012;153(3):515–517.

41. Sullivan MJ, Thibault P, Simmonds MJ, Milioto M, Cantin AP, Velly AM. Pain, perceived injustice and the persistence of post-traumatic stress symptoms during the course of rehabilitation for whiplash injuries. *Pain* 2009;145:325–331.

42. Sturgeon JA, Ziadni MS, Trost Z, Darnall BD, Mackey SC. Pain catastrophizing, perceived injustice, and pain intensity impair life satisfaction through differential patterns of physical and psychological disruption. *Scand J Pain* 2017;17:390–396.

43. McParland JL, Knussen C. Catastrophizing mediates the relationship between the personal belief in a just world and pain outcomes among chronic pain. *Psychol Inj Law* 2016;9:23–30.

44. Yakobov E, Suso-Ribera C, Vrinceanu T, Adams H, Sullivan MJL. Trait perceived injustice is associated with pain intensity and pain behavior in participants undergoing an experimental pain induction procedure. *J Pain* 2019;209(5):592–599.

45. McParland JL, Eccleston C. "It's not fair": social justice appraisals in the context of chronic pain. *Curr Dir Psychol Sci* 2013;22:484–489.

Further Reading

Cannarella Lorenzetti R, Jacques CH, Donovan C, Cottrell S, Buck J. Managing difficult encounters: understanding physician, patient and situational factors. *Am Fam Physician* 2013;87(6):419–425.

Chipidza F, Wallwork RS, Adams TN, Stern TA. Evaluation and treatment of the angry patient. *Primary Care Companion CNS Disord* 2016;18(3):10–4088/ PCC.16f01951.

Index

For the benefit of digital users, indexed terms that span two pages (e.g., 52–53) may, on occasion, appear on only one of those pages.

Tables, figures and boxes are indicated by *t*, *f* and *b* following the page number

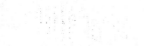